Surviving Triple-Negative Breast Cancer

Surviving Triple-Negative Breast Cancer

Hope, Treatment, and Recovery

PATRICIA PRIJATEL

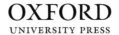

OXFORD
UNIVERSITY PRESS

Oxford University Press is a department of the University of Oxford.
It furthers the University's objective of excellence in research, scholarship,
and education by publishing worldwide.

Oxford   New York
Auckland   Cape Town   Dar es Salaam   Hong Kong   Karachi
Kuala Lumpur   Madrid   Melbourne   Mexico City   Nairobi
New Delhi   Shanghai   Taipei   Toronto

With offices in
Argentina   Austria   Brazil   Chile   Czech Republic   France   Greece
Guatemala   Hungary   Italy   Japan   Poland   Portugal   Singapore
South Korea   Switzerland   Thailand   Turkey   Ukraine   Vietnam

Oxford is a registered trade mark of Oxford University Press
in the UK and certain other countries.

Published in the United States of America by
Oxford University Press
198 Madison Avenue, New York, NY 10016

Library of Congress Cataloging-in-Publication Data
Prijatel, Patricia, 1945–
    Surviving triple-negative breast cancer : hope, treatment, and recovery / Patricia Prijatel.
       p. cm.
Includes bibliographical references and index.
ISBN 978-0-19-538762-9 (hardback : alk. paper); 978-0-19-939385-5 (paperback : alk. paper)
1. Prijatel, Patricia, 1945—Health.   2. Breast—Cancer—Patients—
United States—Biography.   3. Breast—Cancer—Treatment—Popular works.
I. Title.
RC280.B8P727 2013
616.99'449—dc23
2012012425

To all those who have embarked on the triple-negative breast cancer journey, their caregivers, families, and friends. Nobody wants to walk this road, but we can make it easier by helping one another. I hope these pages calm, clarify, and encourage.

Contents

List of Tables

List of Boxes

Foreword

I have been a surgeon for three decades. When I began my training, the accepted surgical treatment for breast cancer was mastectomy. Classical radical mastectomy had been "modified" several ways and a less radical operation, the modified radical mastectomy—complete removal of the breast (including the nipple and areola) and the lymph nodes under the arm, usually with division of one of the pectoral muscles to improve access—had just gained acceptance. We now offer patients a variety of surgical options ranging from lumpectomy (with radiation treatment) through modified radical mastectomy. I can now count at least eleven different surgical procedures that I currently perform for breast cancer: eight on the breast (not counting reconstructive options) and three on the axillary lymph nodes. Surgical treatment is now individualized.

Surgery and radiation treatment treat the disease only in the breast and underarm region. They do not affect any malignant cells that may be circulating outside of this local area. For that, some kind of systemic treatment, such as chemotherapy, is required. Modern treatment of breast cancer is thus termed *multimodality*—most women will get some form of surgery, and some kind of systemic therapy. Many women also get radiation treatment (I will use the term *woman* throughout—men do get breast cancer, and their treatment is based upon what we know about women with breast cancer—because the majority of readers of this book will likely be women).

We've known for a long time that not all breast cancers behave the same. In some women, the disease is relentlessly aggressive. In others, it grows slowly and is relatively easy to control, even to cure. Much scientific work over the past decades has been devoted to finding out how to predict the course of the disease in an individual woman. If we knew, for example, that a woman had a "well-behaved" cancer (what an oxymoron that seems! But there are indeed cancers that behave well—they stay localized, they don't tend to spread, and they don't tend to kill), we could give her less aggressive treatment. On the other hand, a woman with a cancer that has characteristics associated with aggressive behavior could be treated more aggressively.

To that end, in addition to the stage of the disease (determined by the size of tumor and any spread to lymph nodes or other areas), we look at specific characteristics of the tumor under the microscope. Three important markers that have emerged are estrogen receptors (ER), progesterone receptors (PR), and Her2/neu. Molecular "fingerprinting" has identified a subset of cancers that behave particularly aggressively. These are ER negative, PR negative, and Her2/neu negative. They are called "triple-negative" tumors. This book is for and about the approximately 15 percent of women with breast cancer whose tumors are "triple-negative." We see this kind of cancer in women of all ages, but it is especially common in young women. It is also commonly seen in women who carry the "breast cancer genes"—BRCA1 and BRCA2.

The author of this book is a breast cancer survivor whose own experience with triple-negative breast cancer spurred her to research the topic. As many women do, she sought out information concerning breast cancer in general and triple-negative breast cancer in particular. What she found brought out the reporter in her. As a professor emeritus of journalism, she knew how to research and present information. She truly went the extra mile to bring this information together in a highly readable form. As she says, her name means "friend," and she offers this book to other women with breast cancer as one friend to another.

We all hope that more precise stratification of women with breast cancer will allow newer, more carefully tailored, truly individualized treatment. For now, I recommend this book to anyone whose life has been touched by triple-negative breast cancer. Use it to supplement your own research. Because the field is changing so fast, I suggest the following Internet resources in addition to this book:

1. The National Comprehensive Cancer Network (http://www.nccn.com) publishes guidelines for treatment of women with breast cancer based upon best available evidence. These guidelines are updated periodically as new information becomes available.
2. The National Cancer Institute (http://www.cancer.gov/cancertopics) gives comprehensive information about all kinds of cancers. It also lists available clinical trials.
3. The San Antonio Breast Cancer Symposium (http://www.sabcs.org) is an international forum that takes place every year. The latest research from clinical trials is presented. Abstracts are available at their website.

The voice of a true friend echoes throughout these pages. I congratulate her on a monumental achievement. She has distilled a great deal of information down to a highly readable volume. Use this, with the other resources she suggests, as a guidebook on your own journey through this strange and hostile landscape. I wish you all the very best.

Carol E. H. Scott-Conner, MD, PhD
Professor of Surgery
University of Iowa Carver College of Medicine

Acknowledgments

The following healthcare professionals graciously read and edited the initial version of the manuscript for this book. I thank them for their diligence, support, and advice. They encouraged me to keep going on the project, but kept me to a high standard. I am deeply indebted to them for their wisdom, kindness, and true concern for women's health.

Renee Ellerbroek, M.D., is a pathologist with Iowa Pathology Associates. A graduate of the University of Iowa Medical School, she is board certified in anatomic and clinical pathology, with special interest in surgical pathology.

Madlyn Ferraro, RN, OCN, CCRC, recently retired from the University of North Carolina's Lineberger Comprehensive Cancer Center where she was the network coordinator of the cancer clinical trial program. You can enjoy Madlyn's original art at www.ferar roart.com.

Rochelle Kirwan, RD, is a dietitian and health and fitness specialist; she is a program coordinator of the Move! program through the Edward Hines, Jr. Veterans Administration Hospital in Hines, Illinois, where she also works in nutrition and food services.

Carol Scott-Conner, M.D., Ph.D. is a breast surgeon and professor of surgery at the University of Iowa Carver College of Medicine.

She is the author of nine medical textbooks and one book of short stories. Carol also wrote the foreword to this book.

Deborah Stamenhovich, RD, CSO, is a clinical dietitian for the Hematology/Oncology Department at the Edward Hines, Jr. Veterans Administration Hospital in Hines, Illinois.

I would not have found some of these wonderful women if it had not been for the help of two excellent Drake University alums, Pete Brace and Abbie Hansen. I honestly cannot thank them enough.

SPECIAL THANKS to the women who have also fought triple-negative breast cancer and who helped with edits and suggestions from the well-informed patient's perspective:

Noreen Parks is a science and environmental writer who was diagnosed with triple-negative breast cancer in 2004. I tell her story in chapter 6.

Suzanne Kesten is a retired medicinal chemist who was diagnosed with triple-negative breast cancer in 2008. Her *Sue's Escape from Cancerland* blog is at suzannekesten2.blogspot.com/

Kim VanderPoel, LPN, is a Certified Wellness Coach. She was diagnosed with triple-negative breast cancer in 2008. Her blog, *Kim's Ponderings Beyond Breast Cancer*, is at kim-living4today. blogspot.com

WITH GREAT LOVE AND SADNESS, I remember the friends and colleagues I have lost to triple-negative breast cancer in the process of writing this book. While I remain upbeat about the fact that most women beat this disease, I do know it is not to be taken lightly, that it can be a killer.

As senior director of production for Meredith Corporation, Karen Chiavaro often visited my classes at Drake University, walking students through an exercise in which they determined placement of pages in an actual magazine, usually *Better Homes and Gardens*. She was also an invaluable resource for my magazine publishing book. More important, she was a good, upbeat, loving woman who packed a lot into a too-short life. Karen was diagnosed with triple-negative in August 2007 and died in August 2009. She was 53.

Linda Hallam was a magazine editor I worked with when she was at Meredith Corporation. When Linda decided to leave publishing and work on her Ph.D., she came to me for advice. I encouraged her and, ultimately, she went for it. In January 2010, she wrote to tell me she was using my magazine textbook in a class she was teaching in Florida. And, as an aside, she told me that she had triple-negative breast cancer. In April 2011, she was weeks away from earning her doctorate when she died. She was 60.

Neeraja Renduchintala was originally one of the women I profiled for this book. She was diagnosed in December 2007. She quit her demanding, long-commute job in New York to work closer to her New Jersey home so she could spend more time with her two children. I had a wonderful interview with her, but then she emailed me that her cancer had spread. We continued corresponding until she stopped answering my emails. She died in November 2010. She was 38.

WITH ENORMOUS THANKS to my editor, Abby Gross, of Oxford University Press, who encouraged me throughout the bumpy and sometimes circuitous road I took to make this book what it is. She never wavered in her commitment to the book, although I occasionally wanted to call the whole thing off. I honestly could not have done this without Abby—she helped me find my voice and took this book from a dry recitation of research to a series of personal stories that show the face of triple-negative breast cancer; the research remains, but I think it is now much more easily digestible. Abby helped me write the book I wanted to write. Bless you, Abby.

AND FINALLY, THANKS to the beautiful people in my life, who keep me going by loving me, making me laugh, and offering their encouragement and support, especially my husband Joe, my son Josh, my daughter Ellen and her husband Steve. And, for their hugs and sweet baby love: my grandsons Tarin and Eli.

Surviving Triple-Negative Breast Cancer

The Sun Shines on
My Bald Head

I T'S 9:30 ON MAY 16, 2006, AND I AM SITTING AT MY DESK, staring at my phone. The doctor said she would call between 9:30 and 10. I try to focus on a report due later in the week, but my eyes return to the phone. It's like a cobra on my desk and I am all out of flutes. No charming this snake.

Outside my window, the campus is a fresh spring green; students walk by between classes, most in shorts and T-shirts. A beautiful day for a walk, I think.

The snake rings. I check caller ID: *Iowa Radiology*. This is The Call. I get up to close my door so I can talk in private, then reluctantly answer. She gets right to the point:

"Patricia, your biopsy came back. It is positive for cancer."

And so my life is split between BC and AD—Before Cancer and After Diagnosis. It will be weeks before I get worse news: that my cancer is estrogen-negative. At this point I think I have just plain breast cancer; I have no idea how many variations of the disease exist. I do not even know there is such a thing as estrogen-negative.

For the diagnostic report, the pathologist did not test for receptor status; I will learn that after surgery.

It's a fairly small tumor: 1.5 centimeters. "Patricia," the doctor says kindly, "It's not that bad."

I write that down on a Post-it note: *Patricia, it's not that bad.* Interesting that I write my own name, as though I might forget it later. Eventually I transfer these words to the red notebook I carry to all my appointments, writing down data and prognoses, plus encouraging and discouraging words.

This phrase, though, becomes sort of a positive mantra that pulls me up throughout treatment. *It's not that bad. It's not that bad. It's not that bad,* I tell myself over and over. How lucky I was to get this call from such a thoughtful woman. I think of my friend Diane whose radiologist told her that her cancer was so advanced it was incurable and that she likely had less than a year to live. More than 10 years later, she has proven him wrong, but at the time she was devastated.

I liked the radiologist as soon as I met her, which was just the day before. She had a calming manner, even while she made it clear to me that it was highly likely I was facing bad news. "I do not like what I am seeing," she said, and she reiterated that thought multiple times, with a gentle clarity I appreciated: She was treating me like an adult while showing sincere care for me as a person.

I'd started the day with a mammogram, ordered because my gynecologist had detected a lump in my breast during a regular exam. I'd felt it in the shower a week or so earlier, but when I tried to find it again, I couldn't. I dismissed it. I was too busy for cancer.

The mammogram showed a mass, so the radiologist did an ultrasound, which confirmed that the mass was a tumor and not a cyst. I'd had breast cysts in previous years, so up until this point I thought this was going to be a replay of that script. Not so. This time it was a tumor.

She checked it from multiple angles on the ultrasound, trying to keep up a relaxed chatter. We talked about the TV show *Monk*, but we couldn't go beyond more than a sentence or two of dialogue. Monk's oddities were far less significant to us at that time than what was happening on the ultrasound screen. We were all looking at the screen, at the crablike tumor I was growing.

Finally, she did a core needle biopsy and sent me on my way, promising to call early the next morning.

I, of course, hit the Internet when I got home and learned that most tumors are benign, so I tried to talk myself into that being the case for me. Still, the doctor's warning was clear: "I don't like what I am seeing."

So the call is not a surprise, but it is still a shock. Me, of all people, with cancer. I truly and honestly never thought of myself as getting breast cancer. I figured that when I was in my 80s, I would get some form of cancer, as my parents had, my mother with pancreatic, my dad with myelodysplastic syndrome, or preleukemia. Overachiever, I am 20 years ahead of them. I just turned 60.

The radiologist asks me who my surgeon is. When I tell her, she calls him "meticulous."

I write that on the Post-it as well. *Meticulous.* Just what you want in a surgeon. *Meticulous.* This woman knows how to use good words, how to share the positive, how to break your veneer of safety yet help you piece it back together again.

We end the call, with her wishing me well. I believe she honestly means it.

I need to share this news, but Joe, my husband, is not home. He has gone out of town for an aunt's funeral. I am seriously annoyed with him, although I try to tell myself that this is, after all, his aunt's only funeral, and expecting him to stay home thinking about my lump is probably not reasonable.

Reasonable, schmeasonable. I have cancer.

I call my friend and writing partner, Sammye, who ironically was diagnosed with breast cancer a week ago. I was so sad for her at the time; little did I know I would soon be joining her. We talk about the second edition of the book we are just finishing and blame our ill-nesses on the stress of academic work and writing.

So far I am blaming Joe and my career. Not a positive start.

I meet the surgeon the next day. He is a tall, cozy man, and I like and trust him instantly. He has bright, happy blue eyes and a quiet voice and smile. Later, I discover he takes yoga classes with a friend, and that makes me like him even more, and helps me understand why he seems so balanced in such a trying field. Years later, he tells me he drives a Harley, and I am not sure what to make of this news. Better that he takes risks with his own life than mine, I guess. He probably is a very careful driver, though. Meticulous, perhaps.

Joe is with me now, as he is throughout my treatment.

The surgeon expands on my diagnosis: I have invasive ductal carcinoma, or cancer that started in the milk ducts, broke through, and invaded surrounding tissue. This is the most common form of cancer, he says. I will need a lumpectomy plus radiation, and my risk of recurrence is only 4 to 5 percent. I write this all down and think, *This really* isn't *so bad.*

He tells us he'll also do a sentinel node biopsy to see if the cancer has spread. The sentinel node is the first node the cancer goes to; doctors mark it by putting dye in the breast and following it. In the past, women had to have as many as 40 lymph nodes removed, often causing lymphedema, or painful swelling of the arm. If my lymph nodes are negative, I will have radiation once a day for 30 days. If I have any affected lymph nodes, I will need chemo.

He also orders a CAT scan and a bone scan to determine if the cancer has spread to any distant locations.

I continue writing this in my red notebook, which is now decorated with a picture of Venus de Milo. As I write this, five years later, that book is open in front of me. I remember the fear and confusion I felt while writing my notes, and I am thankful for the physical and mental health I now enjoy. Too bad, when I was first diagnosed, I couldn't see five years into the future.

Five days later, the results of the additional tests are in. I have an old trauma in my left fibula, but no big deal. My liver looks good. I do, however, have some nodules in my lung that he wants to look at more closely, so he orders a CT of my chest. And, while we're at it, we're getting an X-ray of the lower leg, to make sure that injury is not attracting cancer cells. Subsequent tests are also clear. The lung nodules, they say, have probably been there for years, but we'll keep watching. We do, and the nodules do not change throughout the years.

I could have the surgery immediately, but I put it off for a couple of weeks to celebrate our daughter Ellen's wedding. She and Steve had been married in Lake Tahoe in March—spring break for her, as she was working on her MFA in sculpture. My two brothers and one sister, plus a niece and a nephew, and even a great niece come from out of town for the celebration, as do Steve's parents. We have a lively houseful, and we have a great time. At one point, Steve's mother tells me, "I can't believe how well you are holding up. I would be devastated."

Huh? I wonder. And then remember: *Oh, yeah, cancer.* I love that I had forgotten.

The reception is wonderful, and I enjoy it immensely, continuing to forget that I have cancer. My husband and I waltz and tango, toast the beautiful couple, laugh with old friends and new relatives.

I wear a gorgeous turquoise silk dress that I had made by a seamstress friend. It shows off my new 35-pound lighter body—I had lost weight in the months before the diagnosis through exercise and diet. I feel extremely healthy, which helps me forget the cancer thing. That is the irony of cancer—you often don't feel you're sick until after you are treated.

I thought I was healthier than I had been in years. I was lifting weights, jogging, eating a nourishing diet. Friends were telling me I looked great. I invariably responded with, "I feel great." I'd passed my 60th birthday with a party and a great attitude, knowing I was thinner and more energetic than I had been on my 50th.

All the while, however, my body was quietly and subversively growing this cancer in my left breast, a tumor so small that when I first felt it in the shower I dismissed it because I could not find it again. I had no family history of breast cancer, had never been on hormone replacement therapy, and I'd breast-fed both my kids, so I figured my chances of breast cancer were low.

Luckily, I was due for my yearly gynecology exam and my doctor also found the lump and sent me in for the mammogram.

MAY 31, 2006. I HAVE THE LUMPECTOMY. When I wake up, I see the surgeon at a counter, writing, in his baby blue scrubs. He sees me stirring and comes over.

"We got it all," he says, his warm hand on my arm. The tumor turned out to be 1.1 × 1.3 centimeters, even smaller than on the mammogram. *Yay,* I think.

And then he tells me I need chemo, that I have estrogen-negative breast cancer. And everything changes. I have gone from small c to big C. When you lose your hair, you look like a cancer patient. And chemo takes your hair. Odd to focus on that detail rather than the fact that chemo is poison and makes you sick. But who says I am thinking clearly? He says I need chemo. That means I am really and honestly and truly sick.

Still, I refuse to believe it and have no intention of having chemo. I plan to go to the oncologist, just to cover my bases, or perhaps to be nice, as I was told I was supposed to do that. But chemo? No, not me.

JUNE 7, 2006. JOE AND I ARE IN THE ONCOLOGIST'S OFFICE. I go in thinking I can talk my way out of this. I can be fairly persuasive, so I plan to explain to this doctor that I really don't need chemo. Good plan, huh?

He is fairly officious, though, and there is no charming him. He is big and burly, and he gets right to the point. No small talk. He tells me that, according to my pathology report, my cancer is estrogen-negative, weakly positive for progesterone, and negative for Her2/neu. I, of course, barely understand what estrogen- and progesterone-negative mean, and I have never heard of Her2/neu. He tells me a negative reading there is good. I later learn how right he is.

He also tells me, "We consider weakly positive to be negative." Later, another oncologist will use the same construction to make the opposite point: "We consider weakly positive to be positive."

I am justifiably confused.

"Hormonal therapy is not an option," he says. I write this down and look it up later and realize he is talking about tamoxifen and other anti-estrogen drugs. He also says "Herceptin is not an option." I write that down and look it up and discover that Herceptin is a wonder drug to fight Her2-positive cancer, which I do not have. So much to learn, so little time to learn it. So little help from the doctor. Did he really expect me to already know all this? Why? Or does that matter to him?

And he tells me that the tumor is 2.1 centimeters. Huh? That's a new number for me—it was 1.5 centimeters on the mammogram and 1.1 × 1.3 centimeters after surgery. Where did 2.1 come from? He insists that is the tumor size, and it means I am stage II. And, he says, the pathologist noted that it is poorly differentiated, a sign that it is growing rapidly.

With a lumpectomy and radiation alone, he says, I face a 35 percent chance that the cancer will recur somewhere else. We can cut that by half with chemo, leaving, he says, "a 75 to 80 percent chance that it will not come back." I am glad I am writing this down, because he is throwing out numbers fast and loose here. Does he really want me to understand, or does he just want to get me to shut up?

He recommends four rounds of Adriamycin and Cytoxan every two weeks, followed by four rounds of Taxol every two weeks. A total of 16 weeks of chemotherapy.

And then, he adds, after this, my chances are 80 to 85 percent that it will not return. A minute ago my odds were 75 to 80 percent. They keep improving the longer he talks. But he does not earn my confidence. It feels like he is badgering me to do what he thinks is right, not helping me comprehend my illness.

He is The Oncologist and I am The Patient. In his world, he speaks; I listen. In my world, I ask questions; he answers. Other patients may do perfectly well with his approach, but he is not what I need.

He tells me I have 100 percent chance of losing my hair—he is right about that—but he also tells me that nausea is "no longer an issue" because of drugs added to the chemo cocktail—and he is quite wrong there. Adriamycin could hurt my heart, he says, so we need to do a scan beforehand to check the heart muscle. And there's a slight increase in my chances of acute leukemia.

I blink. First cancer, then more serious cancer, then a heart risk and leukemia. What next?

He schedules me for the scan and for the first chemo, and we leave his office confused and horribly concerned. Neither of us talks much. Neither of us knows what to say. Oddly, I decide to go back to my office. A good case of avoidance, I guess. Joe goes home and, more sanely, calls friends for support.

I have a follow-up appointment with the surgeon the next day, and he says I am actually stage I, not stage II as the oncologist had said, and that the "poorly differentiated" aspect of my diagnosis is the only real cause for concern. He also recommends chemo, which he says will give me a cure rate of 90 to 95 percent. My odds do keep improving, but my odds of believing the numbers dwindle. As I do additional research, I learn that the numbers do change from study to study, so it is difficult to give an accurate, specific prognosis. I focus on that fact that my chances of beating this are good.

I leave the surgeon's office and once again go back to work, my refuge, where I ponder what in God's name I should do. I call the surgeon for perspective, but he is not there, so I leave a number for a call back. Restless, I go for a walk to the health food store about a mile from campus, buy myself a smoothie, enjoy the fresh air, and try to walk off my nervous energy. I take my cell phone so I don't miss his call, but never hear it ring. When I get back to the office, I see I have four missed calls from him. Clearly, he cares. We finally connect and talk about my options and risks, and he repeats his position: I absolutely should do chemo. His sister died of breast cancer. She did not have chemo.

But the thought of going back to the first oncologist sets me on edge. He may be an excellent doctor, but he and I certainly did not connect. And I need to feel confident with whoever is leading me on this journey. I call his nurse, who suggests I get another opinion. But there is only one group of oncologists in Des Moines. "You can go to another doctor here," the nurse says. "People do it all the time." It turns out that, while there is only one large group, all the doctors within it have their separate practices.

JUNE 9, 2006. WE ARE IN THE SECOND ONCOLOGIST'S OFFICE. He circles the 1.1 centimeters on the surgical pathology report and says that is the size we focus on. He agrees with the surgeon that it is stage 1.

"It's not that big," he says, bless his heart. I understand later that my tumor was comparatively small, but at this point, I know very little, so positive evaluations from doctors carry a lot of weight.

He is instilling confidence—in my ability to fight this, with his help. That is, after all, the way it has to go. I need assurance that the doctor I choose can guide me in the right direction, but it is my body that has to do the actual fighting.

He recommends four rounds of Adriamycin and Cytoxan every two weeks, but he says I do not need the Taxol because my cancer has not spread to the lymph nodes.

Yay, no Taxol.

Boo, chemo. Eight weeks of it, which is better than 16. What a malleable sort I am. A week ago I was adamantly opposed to chemo of any and all kinds. Now I am happy to have only eight weeks of it.

He explains *ductal comedo carcinoma*, telling me that I have dead cancer cells inside the milk duct. My cancer has also broken through the ducts, making it infiltrating, or invasive. "It's on the march," he says. Oh good, I think, John Phillips Cancer.

But he is actually taking time to explain things to me, which calms me, even while his words themselves might be cause for concern.

He also says that my cancer is estrogen- and progesterone-negative, that the weakly positive means negative. And he agrees that "the only thing worse is if it were Her2/neu-positive."

"This is a young woman's disease," he says. Dutifully, I write that down in the red notebook. It is only after I leave the doctor's office that I think, Huh? What does that mean? A young woman's disease? Isn't young good? I like young.

He says my chances of beating this, after surgery and chemo, but before radiation, are at 80 percent. I wonder what they are after radiation, but don't ask, as I have had enough numbers.

Still, he says, it is early stage breast cancer, and that is good. And, while the tumor is small, it is "too much cancer to leave alone. We take this kind of cancer very seriously. If it comes back, it is incurable."

Well, then.

JUNE 16, 2006. AT 10 A.M. WE TAKE THE ELEVATOR TO THE CHEMO WARD. A row of recliners lines two walls, facing one another. Several private rooms open off the back wall. An older woman sits in a recliner, an IV hooked up to her arm. She is reading calmly. A man sits farther down, waiting for a nurse.

A group of women congregate around a friend, chatting loudly and laughing, passing some sort of food around. I try not to get cranky. I do not like noise of any kind, and I have never had patience with loud groups of people. And I am stressed. I tell myself that this woman is going through chemo and I should cut her a break; having friends around her helps her. Still, I am going through chemo too.

I ponder the rules of the ward. What might they be? Be kind, I suspect, is number one.

I opt for one of the private rooms, shut the door, and settle onto a bed, happily antisocial. Joe sits in a chair next to me. A nurse comes in and hooks me up. First she pumps me with Aloxi, an antinausea drug, then it's 10 minutes of Adriamycin and 45 minutes of Cytoxan. She tells me that Adriamycin is red and could make my urine red. That's one reason they call it the Red Devil. Later I will learn other reasons.

I will get a Neulasta shot the next day, to keep my white blood counts up. This is the same process I will follow every two weeks until August. Chemo one day, Neulasta the next. This will be what I do on my summer vacation.

I listen to Ellen Degeneres's *The Funny Thing Is…*on my iPod. Occasionally I laugh out loud and then think I am being inappropriate. I mean, is it proper to laugh in the chemo ward?

The experience is relatively painless, and when we are finished, the nurse suggests that Joe take me out to lunch. It seems like a good idea, so we head to an Italian restaurant and I have spaghetti with meat sauce. Four hours later I throw up the entire thing.

The next day I feel a little nauseated and tired, like I have the beginning of a slight case of the flu. The day after, I perk up and we walk around the lake by our house—a two-mile loop. We end up walking every day during chemo, except for the day after treatment.

A friend recommends acupuncture for nausea, and I discover Abby, who I think is magic. I go to her before each chemo, and she calms my stomach, my mind, my heart. She remains a blessing.

Three weeks after chemo begins, my hair falls out—in chunks. I know women who shave their head beforehand in preparation, but I want to stay normal as long as possible, so I leave it alone, and one morning I shower and pull out a fistful of hair. I end up literally pulling out my hair.

It is funny in a pathetic sort of way.

Joe then shaves what is left. I am officially a cancer patient now. I am bald.

I have a wig and some scarves ready, but the wig scratches and the scarves slip off. I never do learn to tie scarves stylishly the way I see other women do. I wear a liner with the wig, which ends up being comfortable enough; the look is an improvement over my real hair—thicker, with a stylish blend of blond tones. If I wear it too long at a time, though, I get a headache.

A friend tells me that, because I am tall, I would look elegant in long scarves and could make a great fashion statement. I want to tell her to make her own damn fashion statement, but I know she is honestly trying to be supportive, so I say nothing.

My stupid bald head gets cold at night, even in the summer, so I have to sleep with a hat, like something out of Grimm's fairy tales.

I continue working, going into the office two or three times a week and handling other work at home on my computer. Another blessing—a supportive work environment. Faculty, staff, administration, and students treat me normally but expect me to rest, which I guess is my new normal.

A wonderful revolving door of family comes to visit throughout the summer. My brother John drives up from Kansas with Hostess cupcakes, a favorite he and I used to share. Chemo has done a number on my appetite—I cannot even stand the smell of mashed potatoes—but those puppies still taste great. My sister Phyllis comes from Colorado and brings her juicer and makes me fresh vegetable juice every day. She leaves the juicer, and we use it so much we wear it out and have to buy another. My sister Kay comes on her birthday with her inimitable sense of humor. She makes me laugh like nobody can.

Both of my kids, Josh and Ellen, come for a week, and we walk around the lake, visit, find things I like to eat, and just enjoy one another. Both bring books on understanding cancer. Both make me laugh and smile.

And people have enough faith in me to treat me normally, not to coddle me. When I tell my brother Ed I am sorry we cannot go to Colorado and help build a fence on mountain land we share, he says, "Oh, you wouldn't have been much help anyway," in just the way he would have treated me had I not been his Sister with Cancer. He then builds our part of the fence himself, so I now have a thousand feet of wood and wire that was built with a good amount of muscle and even more love.

John asks how I am handling the illness. I tell him I am in generally good spirits, but that I had recently been shopping and decided not to buy any clothes because I might not be around to wear them, a truly unusual thought, but one that does still pop into my head when I am not looking. I figure I have the right to be pitiful on occasion. My brother doesn't give into my pathos. "Yeah," he says, "Better not buy any green bananas, either."

Joe calls my illness "Pat's little diversion," showing his own attitude—this is a short-term setback and we will get through it.

My friends, colleagues, students, and the alums who know of my illness send cards and flowers and stop by to visit, bringing healthy goodies as well as extravagances—café mocha, homemade bread, energy smoothies, and fresh fruit. My favorite cards are those that do not allow me to wallow, but tell me to kick this thing. One even comes with a cutout boot to kick with.

I feel cherished. More cherished than I have ever felt in my life. This is undeniably the blessing of this curse: You learn that you are loved.

This all makes chemo easier psychologically. Physically, though, it is quite a pain. I am seriously constipated, complicated no doubt by my bland diet of bread and cereal and cheese. Natural solutions like walking and fiber tablets help, but I often have to go the chemical route and pop laxatives. I have mouth sores, which I treat with a peroxide mouthwash. My mouth foams like Cujo.

I am extremely low on energy and need a daily nap.

But I insist on being positive—it is my stubborn nature. I'll be damned if I am going to let this disease get the better of me. I am going to beat it, and I am going to do so with a good attitude. Take that, cancer!

On my second chemo appointment, though, my oncologist is extremely late. I have to go to his office first for blood tests to ensure that I am OK for chemo. Today, he is more than an hour and a half late. I envision the waiting room as a time-lapse film. First, a few people are scattered around the room, often sitting in pairs, but usually far away from one another, as though we don't want what the other guy has. Then the chairs fill, bit by bit, until they are all full, with several wheelchairs tucked in. The room is crammed with people, the sick and their caregivers.

I look at a beautiful young woman across from me. She has her scarf tied fashionably. How did she do that? I wonder. She is reading a magazine, seemingly in her own world. I wonder what is wrong with her and if she is as calm as she looks. Another young woman has her head on a young man's shoulder. She has tears in her eyes. Which one is sick? I wonder.

Most of the people in the room, though, are elderly, and clearly fragile and ill. They are accompanied by grown children with worried, grim expressions.

I feel my eyes tear up. This is the face of cancer. It stares at me through rheumy blue and clear brown and blank hazel eyes. Under gray, blond, red, brown hair. With wrinkled brows and smooth ones.

I am one of the sick ones, I realize. That thought and the weight of the crowd oppress me. The tears become stronger until I am softly sobbing. I tell my husband I am leaving; I will wait in the hall. I ask him to come get me when they finally call my name.

A half an hour later, I am called.

I try to talk to the doctor of my distress, but he simply says he had an emergency. Certainly somebody knew he would be that late and they could have alerted us to go out and get a cup of coffee rather than waiting in the room of the sick. He spends his days with us, though, so he has long ago lived with the reality of our faces. But I did not sign up for this. He did.

On the morning before my third chemo treatment, I awake with a palpable sense of well-being, as though I have just been kissed by an angel or touched by the hand of God. Or my mother, who died in 1993. I feel surrounded by love and filled with warmth. I smile. The thought *You're going to be fine* runs through my mind, convincingly. I feel softened and strengthened at the same time, ready to continue this fight, but calmly, meditatively, wisely, thoughtfully. And feeling like I am going to win.

I have my last chemo on July 26. Same process. Private room. Aloxi. Adriamycin. Cytoxan. Ellen Degeneres. Afterward, as I check out, the nurse writes "Finished!" on my chart, smiles at me, and says she is happy she won't be seeing me again. I laugh and agree.

Seems like I should have more of a celebration after ending all this. Balloons. A band, perhaps. Confetti. Instead, I go home and take a nap.

JULY 19, 2006. MY RADIATION ONCOLOGIST DRAWS ME A PICTURE. It's an illustration of how the rays will go into and out of my breast, carefully avoiding my lungs. She sketches it right in my little red notebook so I still have a copy of it. It's a good drawing—not only is she an impressive doctor, but she is a talented artist. Her office is decorated with watercolors she has done—beautiful paintings, calming, showing a warmth of spirit. I love this doctor.

I ask about brachytherapy—radiated seeds implanted in the breast and left there for a week. It is less invasive than other forms of radiation, as only the site around the tumor, where the seeds are placed, is affected. And it takes only a week, rather than six and a half weeks. She looks at my breast and sees that it has healed nicely, making me ineligible—the seeds have to be placed before the surgery heals.

None of my doctors has mentioned the possibility of brachytherapy—I read about it on my own. I am frustrated that I no longer have this option, that nobody presented it to me in the first place.

OK, she says, let's talk about what we *can* do.

She explains the process of radiation. While chemotherapy is systemic, going through my entire system, radiation is aimed only at my lump. It affects only the tissue it hits, and it reduces the rate of recurrence by 25 to 40 percent. I might end up feeling tired, she says, but I will feel better than I did during chemo. I need to keep hydrated and active, to maintain both my mental and physical health.

The fact that I have recently lost weight, she says, will help, as my breasts are relatively small, which will make radiation more efficient.

I have to get a simulation scan first to help the computer match the rays with my site, determining the trajectory of the beam. This will then be saved, and that data will be used every time I come in. I will have tiny tattoos on my chest to use as a guide—these will remain forever.

Five and a half weeks of my treatment will be aimed at the entire breast. One week will aim just at the lump.

I set up an appointment for August 10 for the simulation and then a 3:30 p.m. slot every weekday until the end of September. I go out and buy several outfits that do not require a bra. I hate bras as a general principle, but can't imagine wearing one after being radiated. Ellen, my daughter, goes shopping with me, and we determine that clothes are either comfortable or flattering, but seldom both. I choose several blouses and jackets that are comfortable—loose fitting and of heavy material. They work OK, but I always feel like a dowdy cancer patient in them and I give them away as soon as treatment is over.

AUGUST, 2009. RADIATION BECOMES AN OK PROCESS once I get over the massive machine looming over me, grunting, whirring, sending radiated energy into my body. With my permission yet.

The receptionist remembers me as I walk in, smiles and checks off my name. I go back to the waiting room, take off my shirt and put on a gown, then put my shirt and purse in a locker, and wear the key on a bracelet. The technicians come to get me, and while I am radiated, we chat about shoes and movies and restaurants. I feel like I am among friends.

Radiation really doesn't bother me that much. I use lotion on my breasts, get good rest, drink plenty of water, and keep up my daily walks. I take niacin to counter the effects of radiation, but then I have to fight the effects of niacin—a rush that makes my body feel like it is burning. I wonder if this cure is worse than the disease, but the fact is that I have few of the radiation side effects others complain of—pain, burning, exhaustion.

I continue going into the office once or twice a week and working at home. This has become what my life is right now. It is just what I do.

Compared to chemo, this is a happy time. The radiation department is a place of comfort and calm; it is always quiet, efficient, smooth, unhurried. I talk with other patients, and the conversations are full of hope. We are all on the downward slope of treatment, heading toward home base, almost finished. Some of us are still bald; others have not had chemo and have never lost their hair. The place is infused with a sense of progress that treatment is over and hope that the cancer is gone.

I am almost over cancer, I tell myself.

As I near the end of this process, I begin to plan my reward: two weeks at our Colorado cabin. Usually we go there for much of the summer, but this year followed a different game plan. Usually I miss autumn in the mountains because of school. So I look forward to a new treat, to getting away from cancer and heading to the azure skies and rocky peaks and changing colors.

My radiation oncologist and I often share stories of Colorado. She has recently climbed Mt. Elbert, the state's highest peak. Wow. She paints, she climbs, she saves lives. I am in awe.

I like that I started my cancer journey with a strong, supportive woman giving me the diagnosis and I am ending with a strong, supportive woman sending me back into my life, confident in having beaten back the cancer.

Finally, anticlimactically, I come in for my last treatment. It is September 30, a warm fall day. I wear one of my frowzy cancer outfits, a moss green jacket with a matching skirt with a handkerchief hem. I follow the drill—walk by the receptionist, who says, "Hi, Pat," go back to the locker room, take off my shirt, put it in the locker, wear the key, head to the waiting room, wait to be called to the machine, go in to be radiated, talk about shoes, walk out. This time, though, I get a certificate, showing I have graduated from radiation.

I passed.

It is all behind me—surgery, chemo, radiation. Now, to keep it there.

The next day, we drive to Colorado. Fourteen hours to Pueblo and my sister Phyllis's house, where she pampers me as though this whole thing were a big deal. I keep trying to tell myself it is not, and I will continue with that attitude, as it keeps me going, keeps from feeling sorry for myself or falling into anger.

The next day we head up to the cabin, an hour and a half away. My brother Ed and sister-in-law Gwyn have cleaned it and prepared it for us—windows open, flies vacuumed up, refrigerator turned on and humming. They come and meet us with their dogs Poco, Rosie, and Sophie. We all sit on the deck, relax, and talk comfortably, companionably. At our feet, what is left of our little creek gurgles by.

The weather is with us, like a gift. The aspens are golden, capturing the warm October sun. The mountain is a patchwork of blue, green, yellow, and orange. We take several small hikes—I don't know how much stamina I have and whether I can actually handle the altitude— we're at 8,000 feet. The dry, clean air, though, is easy to breathe, and I walk more and more each day, pleased with my progress. I nap each afternoon, with the sun warming me through the window.

On the weekend, my nephew Russ visits, and he, Ed, Joe, and I try a longer hike, up to a rock cliff where neighbors have built benches to capture the stunning view of the mountain, with the meadow and

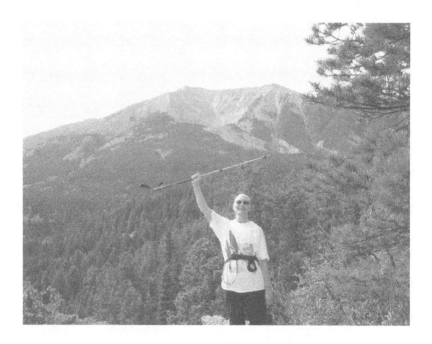

creek far below. It is about a 1,000-foot climb from the cabin. And it is glorious. We stop, gaze, admire.

I take a deep breath to inhale the meadow, the pines, the mountain, the sun, the love of the family that surrounds me. And I give a quiet thanks for the gift that is my life. I take my hat off my bald head and let the sun soak in. Then I raise my hiking pole above my head in a gesture of victory.

Pat 1; Cancer 0.

Educating Myself

Before I was diagnosed, I thought breast cancer was a one-disaster-fits-all disease. I believed all breast cancers were fueled by estrogen and that, as a 60-year-old woman who had never taken hormone replacement therapy, I was not at risk of breast cancer of any flavor.

I am embarrassed by my lack of knowledge at that point. I am normally a curious person—I am a journalist and a college professor, so information is my currency. Yet, I was facing a disease I hadn't even known existed. Like all who are given a cancer diagnosis, I was scared. For me, what was worse was that I was confused.

My fear and confusion were magnified when doctors started talking about the fact that I had an especially dangerous form of breast cancer. (As though I had thought there was cancer that *wasn't* dangerous.)

I hit the Internet and found medical journals that helped me understand what was going on in my body. Hormone-negative breast cancer defied my expectations of the disease. It does not play by the rules I considered normal. I expected it to affect mostly post-menopausal women whose estrogen supplies were depleted. Not so. As women age, they are more likely to get the more common form, hormone-positive. Younger women get hormone-negative. I thought all breast cancer responded to tamoxifen, but found that hormone-negative does not.

The medical books I pored over spent little time on hormone-negative. Still, up to 20 percent of all breast cancer patients—170,000 a year worldwide—have this disease.

I faced a steep learning curve. I had to catch up, and I had to do so fast. And I wasn't finding a lot of information.

Finally, I asked for my pathology report. Oddly, I thought this was a pushy request, and I made it with some trepidation. The nurse did not even blink, just asked if I wanted to pick it up or have it mailed. I picked it up. I had already waited too long.

I read and reread that report so much it is dog-eared by now. I still read it because I am still learning. The report shows how my cancer was evaluated at the original biopsy stage and after surgery. The biopsy showed a 1.5-centimeter infiltrating ductal carcinoma, with Bloom-Richardson high-grade score, which means it was aggressive. The tumor was estrogen-negative, weakly positive for progesterone, and negative for the human growth hormone Her2/neu. The surgery report showed a smaller, slightly less aggressive picture. The tumor on that report was 1.3 × 1.1 centimeters with a healthy 0.3-centimeter margin—there was no sign of cancer around the tumor. It was a grade II on the Nottingham Historic Score, meaning it was mid-range—grade I is slowest growing, grade III is fastest. So the surgical report gave me a bit more hope, and those are the data I focused on. I dissect the report for you in the appendix.

Yes, I was grabbing on to any good news I could find. And I interpreted information in as positive a way as possible. This was important to me—I wanted to maintain the upper hand, to show this disease that I was still boss. I liked to see myself as basically a healthy person who just happened to have a small amount of cancer.

I learned through more research that chemo is actually far more effective against hormone-negative than hormone-positive breast cancer. The potential usefulness of tamoxifen was less clear. Because I had weakly positive results for progesterone, the drug could do a little good. How much was not clear. I opted against it. Enough was enough.

I also learned that the healthy new lifestyle I had adopted a year before diagnosis—losing weight through diet and exercise—was an excellent line of defense, as a low-fat diet and regular exercise are both foils against hormone-negative.

Five years after diagnosis, I am still doing fine. And I am still learning. Things have changed drastically in terms of research. Hormone-negative, especially triple-negative—estrogen-negative, progesterone-negative, and Her2/neu-negative breast cancer—is now a major area of medical research, which is yielding new treatments and prevention strategies. The term *triple-negative breast cancer* first appeared in medical literature in 2005. Since then, it has appeared in more than 600 different publications. So, those of us with this disease are now benefiting from a great deal of new information. We're no longer the wallflowers at the breast cancer prom.

My blog, *Positives About Negative*, has been a learning tool for me and a resource for others. It has also been a gift, connecting me to wonderful women fighters around the world and their loving husbands, partners, daughters, sons, mothers, fathers, and friends.

TRIPLE-NEGATIVE BREAST CANCER HAS HIT MAINSTREAM. Patients now call it by its abbreviation, TNBC. And media reports have changed as well, with more stories specifically on TNBC—although it is often described in scary terms, such as "a particularly aggressive and difficult to treat form of cancer." That maddens patients like me who are fighting to keep a positive attitude. And it is not always true, as I discuss in the next chapter.

The process of educating myself about this disease was difficult and time-consuming. I benefited from already knowing my way around a research paper, plus I had easy access to journals through the university library. I began writing magazine articles about breast cancer, which allowed me to interview top researchers in the field, a serious payoff to my decision 40 years ago to become a journalist. But what about all the other women without the benefits I enjoyed, who didn't have the advantage of that research?

The book you are holding is my attempt to share what I have learned so you do not have to start from square one as I did. Through education, I have learned how to help myself, how to keep myself focused on health and not fear. I hope that reading this book does the same for you.

Here's to our health.

How to Use This Book

For the purposes of this book, I divide breast cancer into two broad categories—hormone-receptor-positive, or those that are sensitive to hormones; and hormone-receptor-negative, or those that are not sensitive to hormones.

I use *hormone-receptor-negative* as the umbrella term for cancers that are *either* estrogen-receptor-negative *or* progesterone-receptor-negative; *both* estrogen-negative *and* progesterone-negative; or triple-negative.

I have chosen to explain and describe this disease through several lenses. First is my story, which I regurgitate early on and use sparingly throughout the rest of the book. Second are the stories of wonderful women throughout the United States—in their 20s, 30s, 40s, 50s, and 60s—who have fought this disease. Several have been disease-free for decades, others for only a few years. I try to present their stories honestly, showing that this can be a harsh disease and that fighting it is no picnic. I focus on the fact that most women survive, but I acknowledge that this disease can be a serious threat. I have dedicated the book to the women I have met who have died from triple-negative.

Third is the research. In most cases, I rely on articles published in peer-reviewed journals, such as the *Journal of the American Medical Association, New England Journal of Medicine, Journal of Clinical Oncology, Annals of Internal Medicine,* and *Annals of Oncology.* I use footnotes throughout; I have learned through my blog that my readers appreciate being able to go back to the original research.

I do not intend this to be a book on all aspects of cancer—just one that fills the gaps other books leave in our understanding of triple-negative and other forms of hormone-negative breast cancer. I still recommend using a reference such as *Dr. Susan Love's Breast Book* or, for a more alternative approach, Sat Dharam Kaur's *The Complete Natural Medicine Guide to Breast Cancer.*

I am not a scientist, nor do I pretend to be one. I have spent five years with my nose in this disease, and I am sharing what I know, what I have experienced, and what others have experienced. All medical information has been fact-checked and verified.

When I began this project, I was thoroughly intimidated by it and often asked myself why I was writing this book and not the people who have researched this disease. But I realized, no book exists, so somebody has to do it. And as I progressed, I realized that I had a unique and valuable perspective, as a woman who has dealt with this disease and as a journalist and educator. I can infuse the book with the voices of this disease; I can show the *who* as well as the *what* of hormone-negative. I can look at it from all angles, the way a patient does. I know when clarification and expansion are necessary and when words such as *aggressive* and *deadly* need interpretation so they explain rather than frighten. I can give readers a sense of control in addition to information.

My goal is to inform, educate, calm, and encourage. Through women's stories I show that this disease can be beaten. Through research, I show how.

The Language of TNBC

Throughout the book, I use the term *hormone-negative breast cancer*, which is a shortened form of *hormone-receptor-negative breast cancer* and refers to breast cancers that are not sensitive to the hormones estrogen and progesterone. Triple-negative breast cancer is a type of hormone-negative that lacks receptors not only for both hormones but also for the human epidermal growth factor receptor Her2/neu.

Most, but not all, cases of hormone-negative are triple-negative. It is important, I feel, to look at the broader range, at all hormone-negative cancers. Because TNBC was named as a subtype so recently, long-term studies using data from the 1980s and 1990s use the term *estrogen-negative* or *hormone-negative*. A good deal of research focuses only on estrogen-negative.

To simplify, I occasionally use abbreviations:

TNBC: Triple-negative breast cancer

ER-: Estrogen-negative breast cancer

ER+: Estrogen-positive breast cancer

PR-: Progesterone-negative breast cancer

PR+: Progesterone-positive breast cancer

I Am, Literally, a Friend

My family name, *Prijatel*, means *friend* in Slovene. Three of my grandparents emigrated from Slovenia and one from neighboring Croatia.

Prijatel is also a Russian word, meaning *friend* and also *lover*. I am, however, not Russian.

The name rhymes with Seattle, a trick I learned from my oldest sister, Kathleen: *Preattle, as in Seattle*. Once, though, Kay had a bit too much to drink and said, *Preattle, as in Chicago*. She no longer drinks.

In Slovenia, the name has an extra *j* at the end, but people in that beautiful Alpine country know what to do with it. Americans are stymied by the name, so I have learned to answer to anything that comes close.

So ask me, and I will answer. And remember that I am a friend.

2

What *Is* This Disease?

FROM THE DECK OF HER HOME IN THE SANDSTONE cliffs of southern Colorado's high desert, Rebecca McPhearson can see all the way to New Mexico, 40 miles away. It's a view she savors, part of a life doctors did not expect to last this long.

In January 1981, Rebecca, then a young mother of three, was diagnosed with cancer in her right breast. She was 34 and still nursing her son, born the previous August. Her two other children were 10 and 12.

Her road to diagnosis was rocky. As soon as she had started nursing, she felt pain in her breast, but doctors shrugged it off. "They said it was a blocked mammary gland," she says. Rebecca, though, knew something more was wrong. It became increasingly painful to nurse, and she worried that she might pass some unknown infection to her son. Six months after her first symptoms, she finally found a physician's assistant who was equally concerned and arranged a series of tests, including one for cancer.

The prognosis was devastating: The tumor had already grown to 5 centimeters and was close to her sternum, so doctors worried that it had already spread to her bones. It was already in eight lymph nodes. Doctors gave her a 14 percent chance of surviving five years. Like many women with breast cancer, she had no family history of the disease.

She was diagnosed on a Friday. By Monday, she had weaned her baby, and by Tuesday, she was ready for surgery. Doctors removed her entire breast and more than 20 lymph nodes. After the mastectomy came more confusion and concern: Her tumor was estrogen-negative, making it potentially highly aggressive. And doctors were years away from understanding this complex and potentially fatal disease.

Rebecca's treatment was as aggressive as her cancer. She had four months of chemotherapy—5FU and methotrexate—every two weeks, from February to June, then doctors gave her a rest to rebuild her white blood cells. After this came six weeks of radiation. In September, she had another six weeks of the same regimen of chemo.

Within a year, precancerous cells showed up in her left breast, so as a precaution, she had a second mastectomy. And her chest wall had been so damaged by the radiation that reconstruction on both breasts was essential to keep her muscle from deteriorating. All in all, she had 13 surgeries on her breasts. She started with silicone implants, then moved to expanders, then to saline in her right breast. Her left breast extender has been in for 20 years and is still going strong. "And it was only guaranteed for one year," she says, laughing.

In 1991 she developed a painful fibroid tumor in her uterus that caused heavy bleeding. It was removed by hysterectomy, and she was given the hormone replacement drug Premarin, which she still takes and tolerates well. Without it, she has miserable hot flashes. That's one benefit of being estrogen-negative, she notes—she has fewer worries about taking hormone replacement therapy.

Through this all, her bones have remained strong, stress tests show a healthy heart, and her physicals now are blessedly undramatic.

Rebecca has always been physically active—she owned six horses when she was diagnosed and continued their care, including shoveling the barn, while she was going through treatment. Today, she still rides the meadows and foothills of the nearby Rocky Mountains. She tries to eat wisely, with a diet rich in fruits, vegetables, and fish. She weighs more than she would like and has lingering shoulder pain from her radiation. And she still cannot stand the smell of Juicy Fruit gum, which she was given to counter the effects of chemo. She still has limited range of motion in her right arm from the removal of so many lymph nodes, yet she keeps riding and caring for her horses.

After her diagnosis, she was worried about seeing her kids grow up, and now she is proud of the adults they have become and the life she has shared with them. Her two older children graduated from Colorado State University and are now settled in their careers. Her youngest—the baby she was breast-feeding when she was diagnosed—survived two tours with the Army in Iraq and is now in his 30s.

Her husband left her two years after her diagnosis, telling her "marriage isn't fun anymore." She was a single mother for nearly ten years, until she met her current husband, James. They have been married since 1993. They share a house they built themselves, a sprawling southwestern ranch near Trinidad, Colorado, that matches the nearby rocks, with a wall of windows and an enormous deck to soak in the western sun.

After treatment, she went back to college, graduating with a degree in cultural anthropology and earning a teaching certificate, plus graduate credits in library science. She has written two books, mysteries based on Native-American culture, using her experiences teaching Utes on a reservation near Durango, Colorado.

Rebecca was a prime candidate for hormone-negative breast cancer, as it disproportionately affects young women. And, while most breast cancers are not painful, tumors can cause pain in breasts that are already sensitive from nursing, confusing the issue and often leading to a misdiagnosis of mastitis, or an infected mammary gland.

As I sit here writing this, I want to come up with a cause-and-effect statement: *Because of X, Rebecca got cancer.* Or: *She did Y, and that's why it didn't come back.* There is no clear cause and effect in hormone-negative breast cancer, though. Yet, some things I know are true:

First, Rebecca is alive and quite well more than 30 years after diagnosis. She is proof that women can survive even the most frightening diagnosis and that hormone-negative breast cancer is not an automatic death sentence. In Rebecca's case, it was an invitation to keep fighting for a long and meaningful life.

Second, not all women, nor their cancers, are alike. Why did Rebecca survive while others with similar diagnoses have lost their fight? There's that X and Y again. We simply don't yet know, but the answer is likely in Rebecca's DNA. There is something in her genetic makeup that made her susceptible to this form of cancer, helped her

TABLE 2–1   The Many Faces of Hormone-Negative

Hormone-receptor-negative cancers can be a mixture of positive and negative receptor status:

- Triple-negative breast cancer: estrogen-negative, progesterone-negative and Her2/neu-negative
- Estrogen-negative, progesterone-positive, and Her2-positive
- Estrogen-positive, progesterone-negative, and Her2-negative
- Estrogen-negative, progesterone-negative, and Her2-positive

fight it, and kept her alive for three decades. Her tumor might have been a less aggressive subtype so her initial prognosis might not have been as dire as doctors thought at the time.

Third, treatment options have improved since Rebecca's diagnosis, so women facing this disease now have more effective chemo regimens, less invasive surgeries, safer radiation, and more sophisticated reconstruction options. This is not to say we have treatment nailed—far from it. Chemotherapy is still toxic, radiation dangerous, and reconstruction often faulty. Yet, we are making progress.

Fourth, cancer changes your life. Rebecca's baby faced failure-to-thrive issues after being yanked from his mother so callously. Her husband left her, and, while she does not seem all that torn up about that fact now, the end of a marriage is always traumatic at some level. And multiple surgeries made cancer the focus of her life for years, during which she had to fight with insurance companies and struggle to make a living while going through constant recovery.

Fifth, you never forget. I was amazed at how Rebecca could recall her treatments—she checked notes for verification, but she clearly remembers her cancer story. How can she not? It was a long, painful process, and, while she emerged from the other end of treatment the same strong woman she was going in—probably stronger—this journey is not one that anybody chooses to take.

Sorting Out the Negatives and Positives

Rebecca knows only that her cancer was estrogen-receptor-negative; she either was not tested for progesterone or did not write that in her notes. Today, she would have been tested for both estrogen and progesterone sensitivity, plus for the human epidermal growth factor receptor Her2/neu, to determine if she was triple-negative.

Triple-negative breast cancer (TNBC) is the most common type of *hormone-negative breast cancer*, but hormone-negative disease includes multiple combinations of estrogen, progesterone, and Her2/neu sensitivity. This is a family of diseases that are distinct from hormone-sensitive breast cancers. As in all families, there is a great deal of variation, built around common characteristics and varying levels of aggressiveness.

It wasn't until 2005 that researchers used the term *triple-negative*, essentially naming a new subset of cancer. This was the result of the discovery of the human epidermal growth factor receptor Her2/neu in the 1980s. Studies on Her2/neu led researchers to a web of subsets within subsets, including TNBC and Her2-positive breast cancers, and refined our understanding of breast cancer as a whole, demonstrating that this is a complex disease fueled by a multitude of factors. The assumption that hormones are the lone culprits in breast cancer was questioned and ultimately found invalid.

This variation in cancer types stems from tiny molecules in cancer cells called receptors. Simply put, receptors make cells sensitive to

TABLE 2–2   Comparative Risks[a]

Increased risk of death from hormone-negative as compared to hormone-positive breast cancer.

- Estrogen-positive, progesterone-negative (13 percent of all cases): **1.2- to 1.5-fold**
- Estrogen-negative and progesterone-positive (3 percent of all cases): **1.5- to 2.1-fold**
- Estrogen-negative and progesterone-negative (21 percent of all cases): **2.1- to 2.5-fold**

[a]Based on data analysis of 155,175 women diagnosed with breast cancer between 1990 and 2001, using Surveillance, Epidemiology, and End Results (SEER) data and published in Breast Cancer Research (2007). Dunnwald, Lisa, Rossing, Mary, Li, Christopher, "Hormone receptor status, tumor characteristics, and prognosis: a prospective cohort of breast cancer patients," *Breast Cancer Research*, vol. 9, no. 1, R6+ (2007).

specific substances. In the case of breast cancer, the essential receptors are sensitive to estrogen, progesterone, or Her2-neu.

To better understand hormone-negative, it is important to look at how it differs from hormone-positive. After decades of research, the relationship between hormones and cancer is fairly clear, which makes it easier to understand how to prevent and treat cancers that have hormone receptors.

For example, we know that the correlation between hormone-replacement therapy (HRT) and cancer is much stronger in cases of hormone-positive than in hormone-negative. Reduction in the use of HRT has led to reduction in cases of hormone-positive, but has had mixed, if any, effects on hormone-negative. And research has yielded effective treatments for hormonally sensitive breast cancers; for example, tamoxifen blocks the effects of estrogen and Arimidex prevents its production. Research on Her2/neu led to Herceptin to treat Her2-positive disease. Tamixofen has been on the market more than 30 years; Arimidex was approved in 2005, and Herceptin was approved in 2006.

BOX 2–1   Common Breast Cancer Drugs

- **Tamoxifen:** Interferes with the activity of estrogen
- **Arimidex:** Lowers estrogen levels in postmenopausal women
- **Herceptin:** Reduces overproduction of Her2/neu

BUT: None of these drugs can fight hormone-negative diseases such as triple-negative breast cancer because they treat hormones and proteins in the body that are not present in hormone-negative breast cancer.

None of these drugs can treat triple-negative tumors, which lack the mechanism—receptors—to attract the substances these drugs fight. The lack of those substances—estrogen, progesterone, and Her2—makes it less clear what actually causes these tumors to develop and grow and, therefore, makes it less clear how to battle them.

So triple-negative breast cancer is a disease that has been defined by what it lacks—and it is difficult to treat a disease based on substances it doesn't have.

Doctors have long known that hormone-negative breast cancers exist, but it was not until the discovery of triple-negative that this type of cancer has caught researchers' eyes in any significant way, leading to a clearer picture of what it is and how it operates.

Here's the snapshot version:

- In general, hormone-negative breast cancer is more likely to affect premenopausal women and those of African-American heritage. It is likely to be diagnosed with affected lymph nodes and larger tumors. Mortality rates are higher than with hormone-positive cancers, with most deaths occurring within the first three years.
- The majority of women with mutations of the BRCA1 gene who get breast cancer are triple-negative, and most basal-like cancers are triple-negative. (See chapter 3 for an explanation of basal-like cancers.)
- Between 17 and 20 percent of all women with breast cancer are triple-negative. And that ends up being a huge number—170,000 triple-negative cancers are diagnosed every year throughout the globe.

Recurrence and Metastases

Recurrence refers to a reappearance of cancer after remission. It can be local, which means in the affected breast, or distant, in the lymph nodes, bones, or other organs such as brain, liver, or lungs. Local is far more easily treatable than distant. Triple-negative is more likely to recur than hormone-positive cancers, but cases of recurrence are still in the minority. In a study comparing triple-negative with other types of breast cancer, 33.9 percent of the women with triple-negative had recurrences beyond the affected breast, as compared to 20.4 percent of those with hormone-positive cancer (see Table 2–3).

And because many cases of triple-negative grow rapidly, if the cancer is going to recur, it will do so in the first three years,

Table 2–3   TNBC by the Numbers[a]

In a comparison of triple-negative and hormone-positive breast cancers:

TNBC tumors were larger:
- The average size at diagnosis was 3 cm, compared with 2.1 cm for all non-TNBC patients.
- Only one-third of TNBC cancers were smaller than 2 cm at diagnosis, compared with two-thirds of the non-TNBC cancers.

Women with TNBC were more likely to have affected nodes:
- 54.4 percent had positive lymph nodes, compared with 45.6 percent for non-TNBC tumors.

The larger the tumor, the higher the likelihood of affected lymph nodes:
- Only 19 percent of women with tumors under 1 cm had positive nodes, while 90 percent of those with tumors over 5 cm had affected nodes.

Women with TNBC were more likely to have distant recurrence:
- 33.9 percent of women with TNBC had recurrences beyond the affected breast, compared with 20.4 percent of those with non-TNBC.

The biggest risk of recurrence for TNBC occurred within one to three years of diagnosis:
- Risk of recurrence peaked between one and five years and dropped significantly after that.
- The average time to distant recurrence was 2.6 years as compared to five years.
- No distant recurrences of TNBC occurred after eight years.
- Non-TNBC breast cancers continued to recur for up to 17 years of diagnosis.

All TNBC deaths occurred within ten years:
- The average time to death was 4.2 years as compared to 6 years for non-TNBC cancers.
- Deaths from other breast cancers continued up to 18 years after diagnosis.
- Survival time from recurrence to death was nine months for TNBC as compared to 30 months for other cancers.

[a]The research included analysis of 1,601 patients with breast cancer diagnosed between 1987 and 1997 at Women's College Hospital in Toronto and was published in Clinical Cancer Research (2007). Eleven percent of those studied were triple-negative. Dent, Rebecca, Trudeau, Maureen, Pritchard, Kathleen I., Hanna, Wedad M., Kahn, Harriet K., Sawka, Carol A., Lickley, Lavina A., Rawlinson, Ellen, Sun, Ping, and Narod, Steven A., "Triple-Negative Breast Cancer: Clinical Features and Patterns of Recurrence," Clinical Cancer Research, vol. 13, no. 15, 4429–4434 (2007), http://clincancerres.aacrjournals.org/content/13/15/4429.full.

with a significant risk reduction after that point. In the study (Table 2–3), no cases of triple-negative occurred after ten years. None. Hormone-positive cases continued to recur for the 17 years of the study, however.

Metastatic breast cancer is cancer that has spread to distant organs. It is more common for an initial diagnosis of triple-negative to be metastatic disease, although these cases are still in the minority—as few as 14 percent.[1] Many of the clinical trials now being conducted on triple-negative are focusing on treatments for metastatic disease.

Recurrences of breast cancer usually have the same receptor status—estrogen-negative, if it recurs, does so as estrogen-negative. But not always: Some cases of hormone-negative recur as hormone-positive, and vice versa. In a study published in *Breast Cancer Research* in 2010, 17 percent of all recurrences changed estrogen, progesterone, or Her2 status.[2]

A *second primary cancer* is different from a recurrence—it means a second, independent case, not a metastasis. That is, your original cancer has not spread; instead, you have developed a new cancer. In this case, you start all over again, and your prognosis is based on the specific characteristics—size, stage, receptor status, and so on—of the new tumor.

Race and Triple-Negative

In general, women of African descent have a good news–bad news relationship with breast cancer. They are less likely to be diagnosed with breast cancer at all, but they are more likely to have triple-negative than Caucasians.

BOX 2–2 **The Impact of Race on Breast Cancer**

Of 2,321 early-stage breast cancer survivors:

African-Americans had the highest rate of triple-negative (28.4 percent) compared with the other races and ethnicities (whites 10.5 percent, Asians 6.3 percent, and Hispanics 10.7 percent).

(continued)

BOX 2-2 **(Continued)**

The majority of the whites (75.3 percent), Asians (71.4 percent), Hispanics (68.5 percent), and African-Americans (59.4 percent) had tumors that were positive for estrogen and progesterone and negative for Her2/neu.

Her2-positive tumors were least common among all races and ethnicities (whites 3.1 percent, African-Americans 3.2 percent, Asians 6.4 percent, and Hispanics 6.6 percent).

African-Americans (average age: 56.2) and Asians (average: 54.8 years) were more likely to be diagnosed at a younger age.

Whites were more likely to be diagnosed at an older age (59.8).

Note: From the Life After Cancer Epidemiology (LACE) Study in Breast Cancer Research (2009).
Source: Kwan, Marilyn, Kushi, Lawrence, Weltzien, Erin, Maring, Benjamin, Kutner, Susan, Fulton, Regan, Lee, Marion, Ambrosone, Christine, and Caan, Bette, "Epidemiology of breast cancer subtypes in two prospective cohort studies of breast cancer survivors," *Breast Cancer Research*, vol. 11, no. 3, R31+ (2009).

African-American women are more likely to be younger at diagnosis, have larger tumors, and face a higher likelihood of dying from breast cancer. And, according to a large data analysis of 244,786 women, published in 2009 in *Breast Cancer Research*, this is true no matter the woman's receptor status. African-American women were more likely to die of both hormone-positive and hormone-negative disease than Caucasian women, regardless of age at diagnosis, stage and grade of the tumor, year of diagnosis, and socioeconomic status. The biggest differences between the two groups came in the first three years after diagnosis in both hormone-negative and hormone-positive cancer, with higher rates of death and recurrence for African-American women. The research used National Cancer Institute's Surveillance, Epidemiology, and End Results (SEER) data on women diagnosed from January 1990 through December 2003 and followed through December 2004.

Some researchers now argue that African-Americans might have a genetically different disease that responds poorly to typical treatments.

Others say the cause of this disparity is that African-American women are diagnosed at a later stage; some tie this to socioeconomic factors.

In research published in the journal *Cancer* in 2007, African-Americans with late-stage triple-negative breast cancer faced a five-year survival rate of only 14 percent. The five-year rate was 36 percent for white women and 37 percent for Hispanic women at the same stage.[3] However, two smaller studies specifically on hormone-negative disease found that African-American and Caucasian women from similar backgrounds treated similarly had similar outcomes.[4,5] The jury is still out on the impact of these studies, but if their results are replicated in larger research, we may have to look at race and cancer through a slightly different lens.

Some studies have shown an increase in hormone-negative breast cancer among Hispanics and women of Indian and Pakistani background, with a higher likelihood of being diagnosed at an early age. Most research shows that Hispanic women and those with Indian and Pakistani roots face survival rates similar to those of Caucasian women.[6,7]

Table 2–4 Hormone Receptor Status Based on Race[a]

African-Americans:
ER+PR+: 44 percent
ER+PR–: 14 percent
ER–PR+: 7 percent
ER–PR–: 35 percent
Non-Hispanic whites:
ER+PR+: 59 percent
ER+PR–: 15 percent
ER–PR+: 6 percent
ER–PR–: 20 percent
Hispanics:
ER+PR+: 58 percent
ER+PR–: 12 percent
ER–PR+: 8 percent
ER–PR–: 22 percent

[a]Based on an analysis of 13,000 breast cancer cases. The percentages indicate how many women from that group were diagnosed with each form of breast cancer. Gapstur, S. M., Dupuis, J., Gann, P., Collila, S., Winchester, D. P., "Hormone receptor status of breast tumors in black, Hispanic, and non-Hispanic white women: an analysis of 13,239 cases," *Cancer*, vol. 77, no. 8, 1465–1471 (1996).

Still, women of all races are more likely to get hormone-positive breast cancer than hormone-negative. That is, when an African-American woman gets breast cancer, she is more likely to get hormone-positive than hormone-negative. But she is more likely to get triple-negative than a Caucasian woman.

The Age Factor

Rebecca, who was 34 when she was diagnosed, fits the standard profile of triple-negative—most women with the disease are pre-menopausal. However, I provide stark evidence that this is another generalization with the usual exceptions: I was 60 at diagnosis.

The reality is that it is more likely for a woman with TNBC to be under 60, but many women over 60 are also affected. For example, in a study of 6,370 women diagnosed with triple-negative breast cancer using California Cancer Registry data, 63 percent were under 60. That means that 37 percent were 60 or over. Yes, a significantly smaller number, but one that shows that, although the disease

Box 2–3   Age and TNBC

Of 92,358 women diagnosed with first primary breast cancer between 1999 and 2003 in the California Cancer Registry, 6,370 were TNBC. Of these:

Women younger than 40 were 1.53 times more likely than 60- to 69-year-olds to be diagnosed with triple-negative breast cancer.

63 percent of those with TNBC were under 60, as compared to only 50 percent of those with hormone-positive being under 60.

The median age of those with TNBC was 54, as compared to 60 for hormone-positive.

Source: Bauer, Katrina R., Brown, Monica, Cress, Rosemary D., Parise, Carol A., and Caggiano, Vincent, "Descriptive analysis of estrogen receptor (ER)-negative, progesterone receptor (PR)-negative, and HER2-negative invasive breast cancer, the so-called triple-negative phenotype: a population-based study from the California cancer registry," *Cancer*, vol. 109, no. 9, 1721–1728 (2007), http://onlinelibrary.wiley.com/doi/10.1002/cncr.22618/pdf.

BOX 2–4   **Tying Race and Age Together**

White women are more likely to be older at a diagnosis of TNBC than Asian or African-American women. The Life After Cancer Epidemiology Study linked age and race of women with TNBC and determined the average age for:

African-Americans: 56.2 years old
Asians: 54.8 years old
Whites: 59.8 years old

Source: Kwan, Marilyn, Kushi, Lawrence, Weltzien, Erin, Maring, Benjamin, Kutner, Susan, Fulton, Regan, Lee, Marion, Ambrosone, Christine, and Caan, Bette, "Epidemiology of breast cancer subtypes in two prospective cohort studies of breast cancer survivors," *Breast Cancer Research*, vol. 11, no. 3, R31+ (2009).

disproportionately affects young women, a good number of older women are also fighting TNBC.

For example, if 170,000 women across the world are diagnosed yearly with triple-negative, as experts project, and they follow the 63/37 percent split, that means that 107,100 cases will be under 60 and 62,900 will be 60 or over.

Race is an important variable when looking at age, with African-American and Asian women more likely to be younger at diagnosis than white women. In fact, the average for white women was just a hair under 60—59.8 years.

BRCA Mutations

The BRCA1 tumor-suppressing gene was first identified in 1994 as part of research on cancer-prone families. Scientists studied the gene alterations that were passed from one generation to another and determined one consistent variable: a mutation of the BRCA1 gene. A year later, in 1995, they discovered a second mutation, of the BRCA2 gene. Cancer-prone families had a higher likelihood of an alteration in both these genes, which translated to a higher likelihood of both breast and ovarian cancer.

BOX 2–5 **Cancer-Prone Families and the BRCA Gene**

BRCA is a tumor-suppressing gene common in all women. Genetic mutations run in families, and those mutations are what can make members of that family cancer-prone.

Both the BRCA1 and BRCA2 mutations are linked to an increased risk of breast cancer, especially triple-negative breast cancer.

In addition, to demonstrate the personal nature of cancer, they determined that the genetic mutations were unique in each family, with each family having distinct genetic alterations.

Ultimately, with the understanding of the triple-negative subtype, scientists learned that most women with the BRCA mutation who got breast cancer got triple-negative breast cancer. Their tumors were also likely to be basal-like. And they were most likely to get cancer at a younger age.

However, not all women with triple-negative have the BRCA mutation. The correlation works one way but not necessarily the other: Women with the genetic mutation who get breast cancer are more likely to have TNBC than other forms, but women with TNBC do not necessarily have the mutation. Likewise, not all triple-negative cancers are basal-like.

And, in an intriguing turn, a 2010 study of 77 women with TNBC treated at the MD Anderson Cancer Center showed that those with TNBC and the BRCA mutation actually faced a lowered risk of recurrence than women with TNBC but without the mutation. However, these results need to be replicated in a larger study population before we draw any definite conclusions.[8]

Nuts and Bolts

Finding Dr. Right

Whether a doctor likes or dislikes you can affect your care, says Jerome Groopman, M.D., in *How Doctors Think*. Doctors who like you are more apt to listen to your complaints and take them seriously, rather than jump to conclusions based on generalities that may or may not apply. Worse, not listening may mean they miss or misdiagnose important symptoms. These feelings can be even more pronounced in the seriously ill, Groopman says. Some doctors have problems dealing with patients with poor prognoses because it makes them feel powerless and frustrated. To get the treatment you need:

Get the best care you can afford. If this means heading out of town, do it. Cancer is a big deal; it deserves the best docs. *U.S. News and World Report* regularly updates its list of the top 50 cancer centers.[9] If you are in a city with multiple options, ask around. I got a second opinion from an oncologist in the same practice as the oncologist who first saw me; I chose the second doctor.

Ask questions. A good doctor will take time to answer them. My radiation oncologist even drew a picture for me, explaining how radiation works. She spent more than an hour talking with me and my husband about all types of treatment. And she treated me like a smart adult who could understand her. A good doctor should be comfortable with you asking questions freely during your office visits. Keep asking until you get an answer that makes sense to you. If, after you get home, things still aren't making sense the way they should, call back.

Find a patient advocate. If you cannot wrap your head around this information, don't try to go it alone. Better yet, go to a center that has a nurse navigator or nurse advocate program—these people are trained to help you make sense of treatment. They ask the questions you don't know to ask, and they understand the answers.

Yeah, But...

The downside of the research popularity of triple-negative is that the media and medical journals have developed catch phrases for it, such as *deadly, particularly aggressive,* or, my favorite, *a lethal triad.* People who write these words do not realize that they can terrify the women who read them, hitting like a heavy thud on our hearts. Researchers are trying to define the disease. Patients are trying to beat it.

The aggressive nature of hormone-negative is a comparative measure. That is, these cancers are, in general, more aggressive than hormone-positive cancers—although, in some cases, only slightly more aggressive. And some hormone-negative cancers can actually be less aggressive than some hormone-positive cancers. Scientists work in generalizations, defining how the disease affects women as a group. Individual cases vary and, researchers increasingly say, are as unique as our DNA.

How researchers classify triple-negative, for example, can be confusing. My own case—negative for estrogen and Her2, but weakly positive for progesterone—puts me in a fairly narrow sub-set. Yet I had two oncologists tell me that they classify weakly pos-itive as a negative, meaning I would be triple-negative. Researchers disagree, usually considering any level of positive as being posi-tive. It is possible, though, that my weakly positive progesterone put me in a less aggressive subset that is so small it is seldom researched.

So let's look at some of the data and what they mean. And rather than simply accepting the gloomy picture that is often presented, let's approach this in the enterprising spirit of *yeah, but....*

It is true that hormone-negative breast cancers can be more aggressive than hormone-positive. *But* the majority of women who get the disease survive.

It is true that most cases of recurrence come within the first three years. *But* that means that those who hit five years are looking at an excellent prognosis. A better prognosis, in fact, than those with hormone-positive.

It is true that triple-negative is more likely to have spread to the lymph nodes. *But* many women with TNBC have no positive nodes—and, if they do, they still beat the disease and survive.

I have learned to turn statistics around to improve my perspec-tive. For example, when research says that 30 percent of the women with triple-negative died in a particular study, I turn this around and realize that 70 percent of the women survived. And I plan to be one of those women. And if, in another study, a triple-negative woman faces a twofold increased risk of death compared with one who is hor-mone-positive, I look at the fact that the difference might be between a 10 percent risk and a 20 percent risk. So a triple-negative woman would then face a 20 percent risk. And, while those decreased odds are startling and sobering, they still mean an 80 percent chance of *not* dying. Even starting with a poorer prognosis, the odds can still be with you.

BOX 2–6 **Encouraging Survival Rates**

In a study at the MD Anderson Cancer Center of 2,838 women treated with adjuvant (after surgery) chemotherapy between 1985 and 2001:

92.9 percent of women with stage I hormone-negative breast cancer had no recurrences within 5 years.

89 percent of those with stage II had no recurrences within 5 years.

87 percentof those with stage III had no recurrences within 5 years.

Source: Brewster, A. M., Hortobagyi, G. N., Broglio, K. R., Shu-Wan Kau, Santa-Maria, C. A., Arun, B., Buzdar, A. U., Booser, D. J., Valero, V., Bondy, M., and Esteva, F. J., "Residual risk of breast cancer recurrence 5 years after adjuvant therapy," *Journal of the National Cancer Institute*, vol. 100, no. 16, 1179–1183 (2008), http://jnci.oxfordjournals.org/content/100/16/1179.full.pdf+html.

Additional Resources

The following journal articles provide excellent overviews of triple-negative breast cancer; full copies are available online.

Anders, Carey, and Carey, Lisa A., "Understanding and treating triple-negative breast cancer." *Oncology*, vol. 22, no. 11 (2008).

Badve, Sunil Badve, et al. "Basal-like and triple-negative breast cancers: a critical review with an emphasis on the implications for pathologists and oncologists." *Modern Pathology*, vol. 24, no. 2, 157–167 (2011).

Foulkes, William D., Smith, Ian E., and Reis-Filho, Jorge S. "Triple-negative breast cancer," *New England Journal of Medicine*, vol. 363, 1936–1948 (2010).

Profile

A Doctor Gets a Diagnosis

Hellena Scott-Okafor wonders whether being African-American was a reason that her tumor went from a small lump to 3.5

centimeters in two months. The Gainesville, Florida physician and mother of four was diagnosed with triple-negative breast cancer in March 2009 at age 44. A month before she found the lump, her breast became tender and painful. She dismissed it. It was nothing. Then she felt the lump. Even then, she didn't have a sense of urgency about getting to the doctor and ended up rescheduling her regular mammogram. She had a history of fibrocystic breast disease and thought the lump was just fibroids again. She was overweight and worried about heart disease. "I didn't think it would be breast cancer," she says.

Still, she had breast cancer in her family—her maternal grandmother and an aunt. But her grandmother was hormone-positive and died at age 96—11 years after her diagnosis—from complications of a hip fracture. Her aunt is now dealing with hormone-negative and Her2-positive.

That history put her at an elevated risk for breast cancer, and her African heritage and young age put her at higher risk of triple-negative. Nobody in her family has been tested for the BRCA mutation.

Hellena was picky about who treated her. She interviewed potential oncologists, making sure they were all working as a team and that they treated her like the wise woman she is—not because she's a doctor, but because she was a patient with a serious illness. "I needed to see if we could connect," she says. "Could I get them to see the value of my life and my views? I did not need it to be a stretch for them to treat me well."

What's more, she wanted to go after this disease with force and she wanted doctors who agreed. "I needed to know they understood the sense of urgency that I had in determining my treatment choices and they were on board with being aggressive."

Ultimately, she chose all women physicians. "They were people I could identify with," she says. And they agreed with aggressive treatment: a double mastectomy plus chemo—Adriamycin and Cytoxan followed by a taxane—and radiation. She opted out of reconstruction.

She and her husband debated whether she should tell potential health-care providers that she was a doctor herself—of physical medicine and rehabilitation. "Ideally, you want a doctor who is going to offer everybody the same treatment choices and be as kind to you as they would everybody else."

If any of her health-care team didn't work out, she knew she didn't need to work with them. "It is okay to fire doctors," Hellena says. "We are so busy trying to please and be compliant, it's not good for us."

And, even though she trusted her team, she still did her own research, e-mailing physicians and researchers across the country. "Women have to take responsibility," she says. "This is your life, nothing less."

Before cancer, she admits, "My diet sucked." Cancer changed all that. She now focuses on eating low-fat unprocessed foods, little sugar, whole grains, fruits, and vegetables. And she's more active: working with a trainer; playing racquetball, tennis, and kickboxing; exercising to an aerobic CD; swimming; and finishing a 5K walk. "The changes I have made are good for me all around," she says.

Shortly after treatment, she attended a retreat sponsored by the Breast Cancer Recovery Foundation in Madison, Wisconsin. " It allowed me to address the rest of my life and put the whole thing into perspective," she says. While going through treatment, she says, her focus was on the cancer. Now, it is time to move on. "I want to live life to the fullest. I do not want to take life for granted any more."

Hellena has four children, who were 8, 11, 15, and 23 at the time of her diagnosis. Throughout the process she focused on them and on her husband, on living rather than dying. She had to counter others' attitudes to keep herself positive. "People label you, pity you. The fact of the matter is we're still living. There is no weakness in any of this."

"The diagnosis and the disease don't have to be a definition of who we are. I can't let it define me. I know people who have TNBC and always face the fear that the other shoe is going to fall and live their lives according to that. I don't think it's going to end here for me. It helps knowing that for this period of time, I was able to beat it down."

She chose to live life to the fullest since diagnosis, which included taking a course in lay ministry at her church. "My faith is a vital part of my life and grew even stronger during this journey. I believe that the joy of the Lord was my strength during that time. I look back and know that I am blessed. It was only by His grace that I was able to be proactive and remain as active and hopeful as I did. I am a wimp and couldn't have gone through that ordeal without Him. I even believe a small part of my motivation to study medicine was to provide compassionate care to others who, like me, are 'sensitive.' It actually helped me endure when things got tough."

Telling her story for this book inspired her to reach out to other women with TNBC she meets at the Healthy Christian Ministry at her church and at local breast cancer events. "I think I have found my voice," she says.

Notes

1. Kassam, Farrah, Enright, Katherine, Dent, Rebecca, Dranitsaris, George, Myers, Jeff, Flynn, Candi, Fralick, Michael, Kumar, Ritu, and Clemons, Mark, "Survival outcomes for patients with metastatic triple-negative breast cancer: implications for clinical practice and trial design," *Clinical Breast Cancer*, vol. 9, no. 1, 29–33 (2009).

2. Thompson, Alastair, Jordan, Lee, Quinlan, Philip, Anderson, Elizabeth, Skene, Anthony, Dewar, John, and Purdie, Colin, "Prospective comparison of switches in biomarker status between primary and recurrent breast cancer: the Breast Recurrence In Tissues Study (BRITS)," *Breast Cancer Research*, vol. 12, no. 6, R92+ (2010).

3. Bauer, Katrina R., Brown, Monica, Cress, Rosemary D., Parise, Carol A., and Caggiano, Vincent, "Descriptive analysis of estrogen receptor (ER)-negative, progesterone receptor (PR)-negative, and HER2-negative invasive breast cancer, the so-called triple-negative phenotype: a population-based study from the California cancer registry," *Cancer*, vol. 109, no. 9, 1721–1728 (2007), http://onlinelibrary.wiley.com/doi/10.1002/cncr.22618/pdf.

4. Chu, Quyen D., Burton, Gary, Glass, Jonathan, Smith, Mark, and Li, Benjamin D., "Impact of race and ethnicity on outcomes for estrogen receptor-negative breast cancers: experience of an

academic center with a charity hospital," *Journal of the American College of Surgeons*, vol. 210, no. 5, 585–592 (2010).

5. Sachdev, Jasgit C., Ahmed, Saira, Mirza, Muhammad M., Farooq, Aamer, Kronish, Lori, and Jahanzeb, Mohammad, "Does race affect outcomes in triple negative breast cancer?" *Breast Cancer: Basic and Clinical Research*, vol. 4, 23–33 (2010).

6. Caan, Bette, Sternfeld, Barbara, Gunderson, Erica, Coates, Ashley, Quesenberry, Charles, and Slattery, Martha L., "Life After Cancer Epidemiology (LACE) Study: a cohort of early stage breast cancer survivors (United States)," *Cancer Causes and Control*, vol. 16, no. 5, 545–556 (2005).

7. Kakarala, Madhuri, Rozek, Laura, Cote, Michele, Liyanage, Samadhi, and Brenner, Dean, "Breast cancer histology and receptor status characterization in Asian Indian and Pakistani women in the U.S.—a SEER analysis," *BMC Cancer*, vol. 10, no. 1, 191+ (2010), http://www.biomedcentral.com/1471–2407/10/191.

8. Find the full news release from MD Anderson at http://www.mdanderson.org/newsroom/news-releases/2010/.

9. Get the list at http://health.usnews.com/best-hospitals/rankings/cancer.

3

Understanding Your Diagnosis

Lynda Harper found her lump months before she finally went to the doctor to get it tested. "I was in a weird state of denial," she says. "I had lumpy breasts and no risk factors." The lump hurt, and she also had itching around the site where the cancer was found, but had never heard of that as a symptom.

Lynda, who was 62 at the time, lives in an unincorporated town in Colorado's eastern plains. And that location was one reason for her slow response—it simply is not easy to get health care in rural America, she says. Small communities lack the resources to keep doctors and to staff clinics. The result is inconsistent care and long drives to see specialists. You may see one doctor on one visit, another doctor the next time. Doctor One may or may not have communicated well with Doctor Two, who likely has a sketchy sense of your medical history.

"In the past, young doctors just getting started in a practice would be recruited and would move here and work full time for a few years before moving on," she says. "Now, more frequently, we have doctors who live elsewhere and travel here to work in the local clinic or hospital only two or three days a week, so it is difficult to see the same doctor each time."

Lynda had faced frustrations with the revolving door of local doctors before her diagnosis. She had not felt well since she'd had gall bladder surgery two years before. She couldn't digest fat, she was constantly tired, and she had a general feeling that something was wrong. She met with several doctors who did multiple tests and assured her she was fine.

"But I knew something was wrong," she says. If she'd had one primary care doctor, she says, maybe she could have pinpointed the problem. But a series of doctors seeing her at different times with different perspectives added up to irregular and ineffective treatment.

Finally, the lump and the pain motivated her to head to specialists in Denver, nearly 150 miles away. Doctors there did a biopsy and, in April 2007, diagnosed breast cancer: a 2-centimeter tumor with no affected lymph nodes. They recommended a lumpectomy and radiation. It wasn't until after surgery that she got a complete pathology report and learned that she was triple-negative.

She went into surgery thinking that would be the first of only two steps, the second being radiation. Then she'd be through. After surgery, though, when doctors learned the tumor was triple-negative, they told her she would also need chemotherapy.

She had been exhausted before surgery, and now she felt a deep fatigue. And she did not need additional bad news.

She had five acres to tend on her own—her husband died in 1986, at the age of 38. And she had to keep working. Not only did she need to make a living, she needed her job for the insurance. Her employers supported her in the way it mattered—they let her telecommute so she could work while she was out of town for treatment.

And she began having what she calls "breast cancer dreams." Disturbing, dark, and frightening. Browsing through an old sketchbook, she found a prescient drawing she had done before diagnosis. Looking at it through the eyes of a cancer patient, she saw an illustration of an out-of-control cancer cell.

Through it all, she wondered if she were strong enough for chemo. "All my instincts told me not to do it," she says. Nevertheless, at the insistence of her doctors in Denver, she had a port installed in preparation for treatment. The day before chemo was to start, though, the port developed blood clots at both ends. Her entire arm was red, swollen, and hot.

She put it all together and decided she could not handle chemo. She cancelled her appointment. Eventually her oncologist agreed

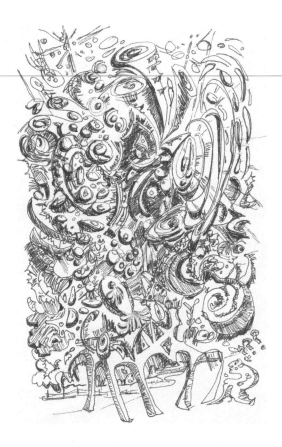

that she probably made the right decision. Hers was a small cancer with no affected nodes—stage I, or early stage cancer—so she faced better prospects than women with more advanced disease.

But she remained exhausted, and she still had radiation ahead of her. She realized that if she were going to fight cancer, she would need to strengthen her entire body, to get to the bottom of why she was so weak. A naturopathic physician in Colorado Springs put her on a high-protein, low-fat diet.

By early June, she felt well enough to start radiation. But she couldn't do it locally. Driving to Denver every day for six weeks was not an option, so she moved to Colorado Springs to stay with her daughter during treatment.

Still, she was fatigued when she started and she was fatigued when she completed treatment.

Doctors told her it would take her six months to get over the effects of radiation, so she looked at the calendar. February 2008. That was the date she would be well. But the date came and went, and she still was exhausted.

"This is the best I am ever going to feel," she thought.

Then she went to a retreat for cancer patients in Arizona sponsored by Living Beyond Breast Cancer and met other women who were taking forever to recover. One was an oncology nurse who'd gotten breast cancer herself. "We used to tell women, 'you are going to have some fatigue,'" the nurse told Lynda. "Then I had breast cancer. We did not have any idea what we were talking about. I kept thinking, 'Why is it so much harder on me than they told me it would be?'"

The retreat energized Lynda—she now knew she was not the only one facing a slow recovery. She came home and started journaling. She began a blog, *A Rural Woman's Breast Cancer Journal*, where she shares with others how difficult it is to find medical care in rural America—the problem of finding a doctor you want, the issues of traveling hundreds of miles to get there with worries about snow or ice, wondering if you'll need somebody to drive you, or facing the prospect of having a mastectomy with the local gall bladder surgeon.

Eventually, her revised diet and new home-based lifestyle ultimately did the job and her energy returned. She believes her problem was with food enzymes exacerbated by gall bladder problems and surgery.

Then, on May 20, 2010, she had a postcancer checkup that gave her the hope she needed—three years without a recurrence.

"I feel different after the checkup," she wrote me shortly after that visit. "Like I'm on a different point in that balancing act between vigilance and worry. Now that I reached the milestone, I realize that my goal used to be getting there. On this side of it, I'm just more relaxed and enjoying each day, and I'm starting to make some plans—something I wasn't doing before."[1]

Testing, Testing

Throughout her breast cancer journey, Lynda learned the lesson common to all those with serious illnesses: She had to be her own advocate. Doctors and other health-care professionals can take you only so far. To really understand your disease and to regain your health, you ultimately need to take control yourself.

This may mean leaving town to get the care you need, or even turning some treatments down because you know your body cannot handle them, because sometimes the treatment can cause more problems than it solves.

This can be exacerbated with a diagnosis of triple-negative or any hormone-negative breast cancer. TNBC is a relatively new disease, and treatment options are being constantly studied and revised. This is not a disease for cookie-cutter treatment.

Our health, no matter our illness, is our business. And it all begins with test after test after test. Understanding those tests is essential to understanding our diagnosis.

When my doctor discovered my lump, she scheduled me for a diagnostic mammogram, which showed a mass growing in my breast—a telltale crablike form that is often the sign of cancer. I immediately had an ultrasound that showed that the mass was not a fluid-filled cyst, but a solid tumor. The radiologist did a biopsy that gave the final diagnosis: cancer.

This is a fairly common progression of tests, but not all women are the same, nor are their cancers, and different circumstances might require different approaches. The following are the most common tests to diagnose breast cancer, and how they apply to triple-negative.

Mammogram

In late 2009, the U.S. Preventive Services Task Force caused a flap when it issued revised breast cancer screening guidelines, recommending that women start mammography screening at age 50, with tests every other year after that, except for women at high risk. The group backed down, essentially reverting to the original guidelines—yearly tests after age 40.

We know that the BRCA mutation is linked to triple-negative, so women are encouraged to have regular mammograms as soon as they are found to carry the BRCA alteration. And those with a family history, even without the mutation, should have yearly mammograms beginning 10 years before the age at which their closest family member was diagnosed.

The fact is that because triple-negative disproportionately affects women under 40, it is not covered by current guidelines. And many women with the BRCA mutation may be not know they have it, so they would not have been vigilant about mammograms. And mammograms have been less effective in finding inflammatory breast cancer, which shows itself through thickness or swelling rather than a tumor.

So what to do? In short, be aware of any changes in your breasts and head to the doctor when you have a lump or any obvious swelling or thickness. A mammogram can determine if additional tests are needed. And don't dawdle—triple-negative can grow quickly.

Mammograms can be either *screening* or *diagnostic. Screening* tests are done as routine checkups on women with no symptoms. *Diagnostic* mammograms are done because of physical changes in the breast such as a lump, nipple discharge, or thickening of the breast, or because the screening mammogram showed an abnormality. Common mammographic changes that cause concern include calcifications, asymmetry, or a mass. All of these will require a closer examination.

Calcifications are tiny calcium deposits that show up as white spots on the mammogram films. Some larger calcifications (macrocalcifications) are normal and considered benign. However, tiny calcifications (microcalcifications) are found in clusters; these are considered suspicious and require biopsy. Diagnostic testing may take longer than screening tests, to allow the technician to magnify or compress the suspicious areas to get a better view of the tissue. Additional testing such as ultrasounds may be needed to complete the evaluation of the mammogram.

Conventional, or analog, mammograms are done with film and are physically delivered from one doctor's office to another and eventually placed into storage. Increasingly, though, cancer centers are using digital mammograms, and most professionals consider these the minimum of care. Both film and digital mammograms create similar images, but digital mammograms are stored on computer and can easily be transferred to a CD. Think the difference between your old film camera and your new digital model. I am lucky enough to get my mammogram minutes before I visit the doctor, and by the time he sees me, he has already reviewed the results on his computer. In some centers, this is not possible, and it may be necessary to have your mammogram performed and read several days before the doctor's appointment.

The benefit of digital information is that it can be analyzed on the computer—enhanced, magnified, or manipulated for evaluation and comparison with previous mammograms, making small new abnormalities more obvious. And digital data can be stored in a computer and easily retrieved for later comparison, so the radiologist can compare your breasts from year to year as part of your follow-up treatment. Digital mammograms are an especially significant improvement over film mammograms for premenopausal women and women with dense breasts.

In 2011, the FDA approved 3-D mammograms, which may be more precise and comprehensive and ultimately replace the need for a follow-up ultrasound or MRIs on suspicious lumps. However, they come with a double dose of radiation, so their benefits might be limited right now to high-risk women.

Ultrasound

This test captures sound waves emitted through a probe that's moved over the skin of the breast. Breast ultrasound is not a screening tool by itself, but it is an important backup when abnormalities are found on a mammogram. Ultrasound can help determine whether a lump is a cyst or a more solid mass that could be cancer. If it's a cyst, the doctor can withdraw liquid with a needle; if the liquid is clear and the cyst disappears, you're fine. If the lump is solid, the ultrasound can help guide a biopsy needle, showing the doctor exactly where to extract tissue to send for testing.

Breast MRI

Magnetic resonance imaging—MRI—offers an alternative method of imaging the breast. Breast MRIs can be helpful as a diagnostic tool in special circumstances, such as for women with dense breasts, the BRCA mutation, or a strong family history of breast cancer. There is ongoing debate about the role of MRIs for women who are newly diagnosed with breast cancer. Breast MRIs can provide information about the extent of the tumor and detect additional small cancerous tumors that could not be felt on physical exam and may not have been visualized on mammogram. Some initial research shows that MRIs can be effective in spotting triple-negative.[2] Several studies have shown them to be more accurate than mammograms in women with the BRCA genetic mutation.[3]

However, MRIs do have a high false-positive rate, leading to unnecessary biopsies, more extensive surgery, and more mastectomies than might actually be needed. The proper use of MRIs in the evaluation of women with a new breast cancer is controversial, and several studies of this question are underway.

Thermography

Thermography uses infrared imaging to detect changes in breast cancer tissue and may be used as a supplement to mammograms, especially for younger women and patients with dense or surgically altered breasts. It is not recommended as a replacement for mammograms.

Biopsy

A biopsy removes a small sample of breast tissue that can be tested for cancer. Biopsies can be performed with a needle or surgically.

In a *fine needle aspiration,* the doctor uses a small needle, similar to that used for a blood sample, to extract cells or liquid from a lump. This can help the doctor determine what is a fluid-filled cyst and what is a solid mass.

A *core needle biopsy* is used when a solid breast lump has been identified on a mammogram or ultrasound. It uses a larger needle to remove tissue samples from the lump. A core biopsy is much more accurate than fine needle aspiration, as it provides the pathologist with more tissue to work with. Each sample is analyzed in the pathology lab to determine if it is cancerous and, if so, what type. At this point, the pathologist may identify your receptor status.

A *surgical, or excisional, biopsy* removes either the entire mass or a portion of it for study. These procedures are performed in an operating room under anesthesia. The tissue is then sent to pathology for testing.

Oncotype DX

This genomic test can be an add-on to your pathology report, or you might have to request it. It can predict the likelihood of recurrence in early stage invasive breast cancer, but it has one flaw: It works with hormone-positive cancers, not hormone-negative. Still, the test might be worth asking for (check to see if your insurance covers it first) because it will detail your estrogen and progesterone receptor status. Researchers throughout the country are trying to refine a similar test for basal-like and other hormone-negative breast cancers.

BRCA Mutation Genetic Testing

Only a small percentage of the population carries the BRCA1 or BRCA2 mutation, also called the breast cancer susceptibility genes 1 and 2—some say as few as 0.2 percent. Still, because of the connection between this genetic mutation and triple-negative breast cancer, the National Comprehensive Cancer Network now recommends that all women 60 and under with triple-negative breast cancer undergo genetic testing. BRCA testing can determine a susceptibility to both breast and ovarian cancer, which is important for your health and for the health of other women in your family. Doctors also recommend genetic counseling if you have the mutation.

Breast Cancer Types: Where TNBC Fits In

Breast cancer can be classified by where and how it develops and by what researchers call its *histopathology*—or what they learn from a microscopic study of cancer tissue.

Historically, breast cancer has been defined by whether it started in the milk ducts or the lobules where milk forms and whether or not it has invaded surrounding tissue.

Ductal breast cancer, or ductal carcinoma, originates in the ducts that carry the milk through the breast to the nipple. *Invasive ductal cancer* has broken through the duct wall and begun to spread. The great majority of breast cancers, including hormone-negative, are ductal—estimates range from 65 to 85 percent. *Ductal carcinoma in situ (DCIS)* refers to cancers that have not moved from the duct (*in situ* means "in the place"); these are usually considered precancers.

Lobular breast cancer, or lobular carcinoma, develops in the lobules, which is where milk is formed. *Invasive lobular cancer* has spread outside the lobules. Less than 10 percent of all breast cancers are lobular. *Lobular carcinoma in situ (LCIS)* has been confined to the lobules; this is not actually considered cancer, but a warning sign for potential cancer.

Inflammatory breast cancer does not usually form as a tumor, but rather as a swelling or thickening of the breast, which can be misdiagnosed as an infection. Partially because of the delayed diagnosis, this type of cancer often spreads to the lymph nodes and has a poorer prognosis than other forms of breast cancer. IBC accounts for fewer than 5 percent of all breast cancers.

Metaplastic breast cancer (not to be confused with metastatic breast cancer) is a type of invasive ductal cancer. It is a unique disease, with cells from other parts of the body such as the skin and bone being found inside the tumor. It is often triple-negative and tends to be diagnosed at an advanced stage with local recurrence; it represents fewer than 1 percent of all breast cancers.

Her2-positive cancer may have a correlation to inflammatory breast cancer; different studies show from 25 percent to 52 percent of all IBC cancers also being Her2-positive.[4] About 40 percent of IBC cancers are triple-negative.

Molecular and Genetic Subtypes

With the discovery of Her2/neu, researchers began going beyond these categories and classifying breast cancer based on the tumor's molecular and genetic characteristics. The result was four broad subtypes, with hormone-negative being most commonly connected to basal-like cancers.

Basal-like breast cancers are so named because they grow in the basal layer of the breast, the outer layer that lines the mammary ducts. These cancers are often triple-negative; in fact, some classifications use basal-like and triple-negative interchangeably. Research, though, shows that the two are different and should not be automatically lumped together. Some hormone-positive cancers can be basal-like, and some triple-negative cancers are not basal.

Basal tumors can be highly aggressive and associated with a poorer prognosis; they are more likely to spread to the lymph nodes, even when they are small. Most cancers associated with mutations in the breast cancer genes, BRCA1 and BRCA2, are basal-like.

TABLE 3–1 Basal Cancer by the Numbers

Of 97 triple-negative tumors compared to 102 non-TNBC tumors at the Netherlands Cancer Institute:

91 percent of the TNBC tumors were basal-like.

The other 9 percent were normal or could not be classified.

18.6 percent of the non-TNBC tumors were also basal-like[a]

Of 496 cases of invasive breast cancer in the Carolina Breast Cancer Study:

20 percent of all breast cancers were basal-like, all of which were hormone-negative.

51 percent were luminal A.

16 percent were luminal B.

7 percent were Her2-positive.

Basal-like tumors were most common in premenopausal and African-American women. Premenopausal African-American women were more likely to have basal-like tumors than postmenopausal African-American women.[b]

[a]Kreike, Bas, van Kouwenhove, Marieke, Horlings, Hugo, Weigelt, Britta, Peterse, Hans, Bartelink, Harry, and van de Vijver, Marc, "Gene expression profiling and histopathological characterization of triple-negative/basal-like breast carcinomas," *Breast Cancer Research*, vol. 9, no. 5, R65+ (2007).
[b]Carey, Lisa A., Perou, Charles M., Livasy, Chad A., Dressler, Lynn G., Cowan, David, Conway, Kathleen, Karaca, Gamze, Troester, Melissa A., Tse, Chiu K., Edmiston, Sharon, Deming, Sandra L., Geradts, Joseph, Cheang, Maggie C. U., Nielsen, Torsten O., Moorman, Patricia G., Earp, H. Shelton, and Millikan, Robert C., "Race, breast cancer subtypes, and survival in the Carolina Breast Cancer Study," *JAMA*, vol. 295, no. 21, 2492–2502 (2006), http://www.ptolemy.ca/members/archives/2007/BreastCancer/Carey_2006.pdf/.

Claudin-low breast cancer is a newly defined molecular subtype that is usually triple-negative and shows a tendency to metastasize. It is currently being researched; definitive information will come from more study.

Her2-positive cancers are positive for the epidermal growth factor receptor 2, or Her2/neu. They can be highly aggressive, with a high likelihood of affected lymph nodes. They are also more likely to be hormone-negative.

Luminal A cancers start in cells in the inner lining of the mammary ducts. These are the most common types of breast cancer and the least aggressive. They most often are estrogen- and progesterone-positive and Her2-negative and more likely to affect older women. It is highly unlikely for luminal A cancers to be triple-negative. Other types of hormone-negative cancers, however, might fit in this category—those, for example, that might be estrogen-negative and progesterone-positive.

Luminal B cancers also start in the inner lining of the mammary ducts. They are likely to be estrogen- and progesterone-positive and Her2-positive, which makes them more aggressive than luminal A cancers. As is the case with luminal A, though, it is highly unlikely for luminal B cancers to be triple-negative, although other types of hormone-negative could be.

Research Bite

Six TNBC Subtypes Discovered
Researchers from Vanderbilt University's Ingram Cancer Center say triple-negative breast cancer can be divided into six distinct subgroups, all of which respond differently to chemotherapy. In an article in the *Journal of Clinical Investigation* (2011), they say the disease can be grouped according to:

- Two basal-like subtypes, which they call BL1 and BL2; these are correlated with cell cycle and DNA damage response genes.
- Two "mesanchymal" types, which they call M and MSL; these correlate to genes involved in cell differentiation and growth factor pathways.
- An immunomodularity type, which they call IM, correlated with immune system genes.
- A luminal group, which they call LAR, correlated with androgen, or the male sex hormone.[5]

Translating Your Pathology Report

Your pathology report contains information your doctor will use to determine your treatment and gauge your prognosis. That is, will you benefit from chemotherapy? How many rounds and what type? Is Herceptin appropriate? What about tamoxifen or Arimidex? Remember pathologists' opinions can differ, and it may be worthwhile to have a second pathologist review the slides of your tumor tissue. Go over your report with your surgeon and oncologist to make sure you understand all aspects of it. Read and reread it, and ask for clarifications of any sections that concern you.

If you had a biopsy before surgery, you may have two different reports—one from the biopsy and one from surgery. Pathology reports differ from lab to lab, but most contain the sections outlined below.

Specimen Submitted

A brief description of the surgical site and procedure done, such as *left breast biopsy* or *sentinel lymph node biopsy*. It also explains when the tissue was received, when the report was issued, and the name of the pathologist.

Clinical History

Your medical history as related to this and any previous cancers. On a biopsy report before surgery, this will explain why the test was done, with a notation such a *density* or *palpable lump*. A surgical report will refer to why the surgery was done, often with a simple reference, such as *left breast cancer*. It may also explain your surgery—*mastectomy* or *partial mastectomy*, for example.

Diagnosis

A summary of the pathologist's final opinion about the tumor; for example, *infiltrating ductal carcinoma* or *ductal carcinoma in situ*.

Macroscopic

A general description of the findings based on an inspection of the tissue before it was examined under the microscope. This section specifies:

Specimen type: how the specimen was taken, such as *core biopsy* or *excisional biopsy*.

Lymph node tests: whether they were done and how many nodes were removed.

Size of the entire surgical specimen.

Laterality: whether the affected breast was right or left.

Tumor site: which part of the breast was involved.

Microscopic

What the pathologist saw through the microscope. This includes:

Tumor size: A three-dimensional measurement of the invasive component. Tumors are measured in centimeters (cm). Tumors under 2 cm (or 0.8 inches) are usually considered "early stage breast cancer." At 1.3 cm, my tumor was half an inch in width.

Histologic type: The cell type of the tumor—*ductal* or *lobular*. This also describes the growth pattern: If the cells fill the duct, the pattern is *solid*; if the cells grow in fingers the pattern is *papillary*. The presence or absence of damaged and dying cells, or *necrosis*, may also be included; this can be a sign of more aggressive disease.

Histologic grade: How abnormal the cells look, which is a measure of tumor aggressiveness. Pathologists use two methods for describing tumor grade; the Bloom-Richardson Scale and the Nottingham Histologic Score.

The *Bloom-Richardson scale* divides tumors into low, intermediate, and high grade. Low grade means the cells look almost normal

TABLE 3–2   Tests of Tumor Aggressiveness

Bloom-Richardson Scale:

    Low grade or well differentiated: less aggressive; cells appear almost normal; slow-growing.

    High grade or poorly differentiated: most aggressive; cells highly abnormal; fast-growing.

The Nottingham Histologic Score:

    Grade I: 1–5 points; slow-growing.

    Grade II: 6–7 points; growing at a medium pace.

    Grade III: over 8 points; rapidly growing.

---

and are less aggressive, while high grade means the cells look less like normal cells and are probably more aggressive and fast-growing. The pathologist might also use the term *poorly differentiated*, which is another way of saying high grade, or *well differentiated*, which means low grade. Normal cells follow a clear pattern; cancer cells do not. Triple-negative cancers tend to be high grade.

The *Nottingham Histologic Score* rates the tumor numerically based on its "mitotic" count, or how rapidly it appears to be dividing and growing. A grade I tumor has between 1 and 5 points and is slow-growing. A grade II has between 6 and 7 points and is growing at a medium pace. A grade III is over 8 points and is rapidly growing. Triple-negative cancers tend to be grade III.

Extent of Invasion

This section provides the final staging information, although staging is becoming less important, as other biological aspects of the disease—such as whether or not it is basal-like—take precedence.

Primary tumor: The tumor's description in terms of size and stage. For instance, T1 is 1 to 2 centimeters. The T stands for tumor, and 1 means that the tumor was less than 2 cm. This is an early stage tumor. T2 means the tumor is more than 2 but less than 5 cm; T3 is more than 5 cm; and T4 is any size that grows into the chest wall or skin, common with inflammatory breast cancer.

Lymph nodes: A measurement of the number of lymph nodes that were examined and determined to be positive for cancer. A positive lymph node means that cancer was found in the lymph node. A negative node means cancer has not spread to the lymph node. The pathologist will also specify in millimeters or centimeters how much cancer is seen in each lymph node and whether the tumor extends outside the lymph nodes into the surrounding tissue. A staging of N0 means that there is no regional lymph node metastasis greater than 0.2 mm. N stands for *nodes*, and 0 means that no nodes—or zero nodes—were affected. N1 means cancer has spread to 1–3 nodes; in N2, it has spread to 4–9 nodes; N3 cancer has spread to more than 10. Spread to the lymph nodes is more common in triple-negative breast cancer.

Distant metastasis: Any spread to a site outside the breast. If no distant tissue was tested, the report will indicate that metastasis or spread is unknown. In this case, pMX means the pathologist cannot comment on any spread to another part of the body. M stands for *metastasis*, and the X means *unknown*. If spread is found, the X will be replaced by the number of affected sites found. If the doctor orders additional tests, such as X-rays and CT scans, as my surgeon did, and finds no distant metastases, the stage becomes M0. A stage M1 means cancer has spread to other organs; this becomes stage IV, or metastatic breast cancer.

Margins: The amount of normal tissue that was removed with the tumor. Uninvolved or clear margins mean that the cancer was completely removed. The distance to the closest margin is usually provided. This is an especially important number because clear margins offer a positive prognosis.

Lymphatic (small vessel) invasion: Whether the tumor cells have invaded into the lymph system or blood vessels.

Microcalcifications: If calcifications were seen in the tissue and whether or not they are associated with the cancer. This is important when the cancer was detected on a mammogram with calcifications. You'll especially want to pay attention to this in follow-up

---

TABLE 3–3   Stages of Breast Cancer

Some common staging designations:[a]

T1, N0, M0: The tumor is less than 2 centimeters, with no affected lymph nodes, and no distant metastases. This is early stage, or stage I cancer.

T2, N1, M0: The tumor is larger than 2 cm, but less than 5, with 1–3 affected lymph nodes, and no distant metastases. Affected lymph nodes makes this stage II, even with a relatively small tumor. A T2 tumor with no affected nodes is often still considered early stage, or stage I.

T3, N2, M0: The tumor is larger than 5 cm, with 4–9 affected nodes and no distant metastases. This is stage III.

T3, N1, M1: The tumor is larger than 5 cm, with 1–3 affected nodes. It has spread to a distant organ. The M1 designation makes this stage IV, or metastatic breast cancer.

---

[a]The American Cancer Society has a comprehensive explanation and illustration of staging levels at http://www.cancer.org/cancer/breastcancer/detailedguide/breast-cancer-staging.

mammograms, as clusters of small calcifications can mean that cancer is growing.

Receptors

A measure by the pathologist of whether the tumor has receptors for estrogen, progesterone, or Her2/neu, using a system that stains the tumor after a biopsy. This can be described as positive or negative.

Some labs will also give a level of receptors or quantify the result. Quantification is ideal, because it's more comprehensive. The more hormone receptors that are present, the more likely the cancer is to react to hormonal treatment. The level of receptors may be scored with a 3-point system, with a score a 0 meaning none of the cells in the biopsy sample contained receptors, and a 3 meaning most cells contained receptors. A 2 is usually considered weakly positive. Other labs may simply indicate a percentage, with 0 percent meaning no hormones were present and 100 percent meaning all cells in the sample had receptors. In this case, anything under 50 percent is usually weakly positive. This is the method my lab used, so I was told only that I had some progesterone receptors, but less than 50 percent.

Her2/neu: A measurement of the human epidermal growth receptors, or Her2/neu receptors, in the cells. Two different tests measure this:

Fluorescence in situ hybridization (FISH) is a genetic test that compares the number of Her2 genes to normal genes. More than two Her2 genes for each normal gene indicates a cancer that is Her2-positive.

Immunohistochemistry (IHC) is a protein test measuring the amount of Her2 protein on the surface of the cancer cells. A score of 3 means a Her2-positive cancer. A score of 2, to some pathologists, is inconclusive; they suggest doing the test over. A score of 0 to 1 means Her2-negative.

Nuts and Bolts

Get Organized: Keep Your Records Straight
You're reeling from your diagnosis and you're confused, stressed, worried, and any number of other negative emotions. You have

a lot to learn, to digest, to comprehend, to accept. Don't try to understand it all at once, but make sure you keep your records and take thorough notes.

The equipment you'll need:

- File folders for the masses of paper you'll collect. I found that two-pocket folders worked best, giving me room for my expanding supply of reports while being small enough to keep things accessible. I had one folder for medical records and one for bills and insurance payments (ack!). An expandable folder with tabs will allow you to keep all records together. Your doctor will give you a folder, but it usually is not big enough.
- A small notebook to take notes during medical visits. Get one that will fit in your purse so it is always with you. Write down the essential information every medical professional gives you so you can research it later. Don't think you're going to remember everything. Or anything. Remember, though, to always ask questions while you're in the office—the notebook is there for you to use to research the questions that did not occur to you during the visit.
- A larger notebook, graph paper, or a spreadsheet on your computer to keep track of expenses. It will all seem less confusing and oppressive if you write down a bill as soon as you get it, leaving space for insurance payments, if any.

What you'll collect:

- Your pathology report. Get it as soon as you are diagnosed. You might end up with two, as I did—one after the original biopsy, one after surgery.
- Your blood work. You will have blood taken so often you'll want to try out for the next *Twilight* movie. Keep them all so you can assess your progress.
- Medical bills and insurance reports. Ugh.
- Copies of additional medical tests: reports of X-rays, MRIs, bone scans, or any additional workups your physician might order.

Remember Supporters: I got so many wonderful cards and notes that I needed a box for them all. I ended up putting them in gift bags, and I kept them nearby to reread during and after treatment. I sent thank-you notes to show my appreciation to those who gave special gifts and gestures. Thanking people took me outside myself and was great therapy, in addition to being decent manners.

Profile

A Double Survivor

Pat Jones refuses to believe that hormone-negative breast cancer is automatically lethal, and she provides more than 25 years of experience to prove it. In 1987, she was diagnosed at age 39 with a 1.6-cm estrogen-negative and progesterone-negative tumor with no affected lymph nodes; she had a lumpectomy and radiation and went on with her life, raising her two daughters and enjoying running and hiking in the Berkshires near her western Massachusetts home. As a young mother with two children—her daughters were 12 and 13—she was especially eager to return to normalcy. And, because she had no information to the contrary, she saw hormone-negative as a good thing, as it meant she did not to have take tamoxifen, so she had none of its side effects.

She was cancer-free for 16 years until 2003. She was putting the finishing touches on the dream house she had just renovated and punctured her breast when moving a chair. She developed a hematoma and discovered a lump behind it.

History had repeated itself. She had a second primary cancer—a new cancer, not a recurrence—in the other breast, this time a 2-cm triple-negative tumor. She opted for a bilateral mastectomy—the removal of both breasts. Like her first tumor, this one was node-negative. She's outlived that cancer for more than nine years.

She didn't have chemotherapy either time—her doctor did not suggest it with her first diagnosis and she declined it the second time. Losing both breasts was the easy decision because the radiation she'd had for the first cancer left her breast so sensitive she could not even sleep on her stomach.

The worst part of her journey, however, came when her 34-year-old daughter, Candy, was also diagnosed with TNBC six months after Pat's second diagnosis.

"That was devastating to me," Pat says. "It flipped me out."

Candy caught her tumor early, and it was still small—1.6 cm, with no affected nodes. She also had a bilateral mastectomy, plus chemo—four rounds of Adriamycin and Cytoxan. Taxol was not recommended.

Candy just finished a 10K race and, Pat says, "She is the picture of health." She is more than ten years past diagnosis.

Pat's mother died at 51 of pancreatic cancer, but there had been no history of breast cancer until Pat's diagnosis. Neither Pat nor Candy has been tested for the BRCA mutation. "What is it going to prove?" Pat asks. "Lets face it, we have some variation of some gene. But is knowing whether we have BRCA going to give me and my grandchildren assurance they are not going to get breast cancer?"

Pat no longer runs, but she walks with weights. She watches what she eats, avoids preservatives, and honors her Italian roots with a glass of wine a day. And she has become much more spiritual since her first diagnosis.

As to why she fought off this disease not once, but twice, she says the answer might eventually come as researchers learn more about different types of triple-negative.

"Some have to be less life-threatening than others," she says.

Her philosophy: "None of us is going to get out of here alive. Both the worst and the best come out of a tragedy. For me, cancer made me realize how short life is and how important it is to take one day at a time. I wake up every day and say, 'It is a good day today.' I cannot look at tomorrow. I cannot look behind. I only have today."

Notes

1. Find Lynda's blog at http://ruralwomen.wordpress.com/.
2. Wang, Carolyn, Rogers, James, Schilling, Kathy, MacDonald, Lawrence, and Haseley, David, "Characterization of

18-fluorodeoxyglucose (FDG) uptake in triple-negative and triple-positive breast cancers with positron emission mammography," *Journal of Nuclear Medicine*, vol. 51, 1073+ (2010).

3. Klijn, Jan G. M., "Early diagnosis of hereditary breast cancer by magnetic resonance imaging: what is realistic?" *Journal of Clinical Oncology*, vol. 28, no. 9, 1441–1445 (2010). Find a full copy of the research at http://jco.ascopubs.org/content/28/9/1441.full.

4. Parton, M., "High incidence of HER-2 positivity in inflammatory breast cancer," *The Breast*, vol. 13, no. 2, 97–103 (2004).

5. Lehmann, Brian D., Bauer, Joshua A., Chen, Xi, Sanders, Melinda E., Chakravarthy, Bapsi, Shyr, Yu, and Pietenpol, Jennifer A.," Identification of human triple-negative breast cancer subtypes and preclinical models for selection of targeted therapies," *Journal of Clinical Investigation*, vol. 121, no. 7, 2750–2767 (2011), http://www.jci.org/articles/view/45014.

4

The Biology of Triple-Negative

MELODY WASSON FEARED HER CHILDBEARING YEARS WERE BEHIND her before she even turned 30. Chemotherapy for triple-negative breast cancer had caused chemopause, or the shutdown of her ovaries, which can happen with premenopausal women. But, two and a half years after her diagnosis, she posted new photos on her blog, *My Fight Against Breast Cancer*—ultrasound images of her baby due the following September.[1]

Melody's family history pointed to a good chance of cancer, so she had been vigilant. Her mother has been diagnosed when she was 35, which led Melody to start getting mammograms at 25, ten years before her mom's diagnosis. And, in July 2008, when she was only 28, she felt a lump; she had a regular mammogram already scheduled, which caught the tumor early. It was relatively small—2.2 centimeters—and had not spread to her lymph nodes.

She had a two-year-old daughter at the time of diagnosis and was warned that chemotherapy could mean that she would never have more children. Wisely, she and husband Ryan counted their blessings—they had one another and their daughter, and if that was as big as their family got, that was OK. Yet, exactly a year after her diagnosis, her periods resumed; a year and a half after that, baby number two was on its way.

After she was diagnosed, she went for genetic testing and discovered that she had the BRCA genetic mutation. She had thought of being tested before she was even diagnosed, but she put it off because she wanted more kids and was afraid of the results. In fact, her mammogram was part of pre-pregnancy planning to make sure she faced no hurdles. She found the lump two weeks before the mammogram was scheduled.

Melody's mother actually had two incidents of breast cancer, months apart, with different hormone status. Her original diagnosis in 1985 was of hormone-receptor positive cancer. She had a mastectomy but no radiation or chemo. Five months later she had a second cancer in the other breast, this one estrogen- and progesterone-receptor negative. "They didn't have TNBC back then, but it more than likely was triple-negative," Melody says.

Her mother was never tested for the BRCA mutation. "To me, it is evident that if I had the gene, she had to have the gene," Melody says. Melody's maternal grandmother died of breast cancer, but Melody's two sisters remain cancer-free.

Even though her tumor was small, she had a bilateral mastectomy—removal of both breasts—because of the BRCA tests. Treatment consisted of dose-dense Adriamycin, Cytoxan, and Taxol, then radiation. Doctors recommend a full hysterectomy by 35.

After that came reconstructive surgery. "I now have better boobs than I had before," she says. "You could not tell I ever had breast cancer by looking. I am comfortable going out in a bikini."

Her vigilance, she thinks, may have saved her life. "I think being proactive made a very big difference in my outcome," she says. "I was blessed with an oncologist who believed I would survive and did everything in his power to ensure that is exactly what happened." She opted to go to St. Louis for chemo because of more specialized options than in her hometown of Springfield, Missouri.

Melody strives to help other young cancer patients in the hopes that they will find their cancer early and be able to fight it. She has become part of the "BRCA Pack," people who have the BRCA genetic mutation and are interested in helping educate others about hereditary breast and ovarian cancer.

"Doctors write you off if you are young and have no history of breast cancer," Melody says. "I have met so many young women who find a lump, but think they're too young to have breast cancer. Their doctors tell them it's probably benign, and say, 'let's wait,' until it's the size of a baseball. If a woman has no history of breast cancer, she might not be too educated about it. And why would she be?"

She's comfortable showing her reconstruction to other women, perhaps reducing their anxiety and educating them on their options. Part of her campaign of awareness begins with her own little daughter. "She has a 50–50 chance of having the gene herself," she says. "I think it is very important for her to see me being comfortable with myself and the way that I look. She might have to face the same thing herself."

Risks, Correlations, and Exceptions

A correlation or association means that two things often occur together. The BRCA gene and African ancestry are both correlated with triple-negative. Yet that is far from a cause. Many with the mutation never get cancer at all. And many without the mutation get TNBC. Likewise, not all African-American women with breast cancer get hormone-receptor-negative, and most do not get cancer of any sort.

Melody had the BRCA mutation and got TNBC at a very young age—28. Having the mutation meant that she did not have the defenses against breast cancer that other women have. To be clear, the BRCA gene in its normal form is actually a good thing, a protection against cancer. It is the *mutation* of the gene that causes problems, that reduces that protection.

But why did Melody's body develop cancer in the first place? Nobody knows for sure. It's a puzzle, and anybody looking for easy answers is certain to be disappointed.

Those of us fixated on beating our own cancer want to talk about a specific cause—and a cure. It can be frustrating, then, when researchers talk about correlations and associations instead of causes. But these correlations may eventually lead to an understanding of the cause of this disease. What is there about being African American that puts a woman at risk? How is the BRCA mutation involved? These are huge questions and, bit by bit, researchers are finding their way toward the answers.

The bottom line is we don't know what causes hormone-receptor-negative breast cancer. All we really understand at this point is that it is a unique disease with unique characteristics. Still, knowing how it is different—and knowing that researchers are zeroing in on those differences—gives me a sense of hope. No, I don't feel I can say, "Here's the reason I got sick." I do feel, though, that knowing at least a little of what makes this disease tick makes it seem less ominous. And hidden in its biology are clues to my own biology—and, perhaps, an ultimate answer to why I got sick in this particular way.

When we are diagnosed with breast cancer, we often think: *What did I do wrong?* We question past infections, blame our nightly glasses of wine, wonder about our genes, wish we had lost weight or exercised more, and, in general, stay awake nights worrying about what we did to cause our cancer, what we can do to get rid of it, and how we can keep it from recurring.

I have my own concerns about what caused it—too much stress calmed by too many martinis and bad eating. I had been overweight, and my immune system was shot, as evidenced by frequent urinary tract infections. After studying this disease for most of the six years since I was diagnosed, I now know that the reality of why I got this cancer has to do with a complex interaction of internal and external factors that could be unique to me.

I no longer beat myself up over what I might have done to cause this disease (well, not all that often), but I am doing all I can to keep it from returning. Understanding some of what influences hormone-negative breast cancer helps us understand our own form of the disease and gives us some hints on what we might be able to do to keep this unwanted visitor from coming by again.

The Implications of a Weakened Immune System

The immune system is one of your body's guards against cancer, so when it is weakened for whatever reason, your body becomes more susceptible to cancer and other diseases. A weakened immune system does not cause cancer—it just does not help prevent it in the way a strong system can.

Your immune system is a network of cells, tissue, and organs such as the thymus, spleen, and bone marrow. Acting like your own internal army, it fends off foreign invaders. The immune system can tell which cells belong in your body and which are there to cause trouble, and it is designed to reject those that do not belong. Antibodies created in the immune system target foreign cells, or antigens. We all have a unique antibody profile, again pointing to the unique nature of this disease and the unique way in our bodies react to cancer antigens.

Most immune cells are created as stem cells in the bone marrow; they circulate throughout the body through the blood stream and the lymphatic system, which includes the lymph nodes.

Sometimes, though, the body's immune system is overworked or malfunctioning and cannot fend off diseases. That may be one reason why one person in a family gets sick while the others don't—the immune systems are working differently.

Cancer grows in stem cells and in their intermediaries, or progenitor cells. Both stem cells and progenitor cells cause cell growth and differentiation, but progenitor cells are more targeted and can duplicate themselves a limited number of times, whereas stem cells can divide indefinitely. Recent studies on mice show that TNBC is more likely to grow in progenitor cells than in stem cells, which may ultimately be a key to understanding the origins of this disease.[2]

Once cancer is formed, it can move through the body in the same way immune cells do—in the bloodstream and the lymphatic system and into lymph nodes clustered in the armpits, neck, groin, and abdomen. Breast cancers typically move to the armpit nodes first.

A strong immune system, though, can reduce or prevent this growth and spread, regulating the creation of lymphocytes, or white blood cells, which fight disease. But our immune system can be weakened by, among other factors, poor diet, stress, allergens in the environment, viral and bacterial infections, exposure to toxins such as radiation, too much alcohol, and aging.

Signs that your immune system might not be working as well as it should are frequent colds and infections, especially if they do not heal; asthma and allergies; and fatigue. Many cases of a compromised immune system, though, have no obvious symptoms.

Research Bite

A Marker of Aggressive Disease

High levels of the nuclear protein Ki-67 were associated with higher rates of recurrence and lower survival for triple-negative patients, according to research in the journal *Breast Cancer*

Research (2011). And low levels signaled a less aggressive form of the disease. Researchers say this could lead to two separate subgroups of TNBC with significantly different levels of aggressiveness and prognosis. The research focused on 105 patients who received neoadjuvant (before surgery) Adriamycin and Cytoxan.[3]

Our Genetic Code

Cancer represents a breakdown in our DNA, or our genetic code. It is the result of mutations or alterations, many of which are inherited through our families. Some breaks in this code, though, have no clear cause.

DNA—deoxyribonucleic acid—contains the information on our individual hereditary characteristics and the genetic instructions that make us who we are and keep us healthy. The human DNA has 20,000 to 25,000 genes, so when you get frustrated that we still know so little about cancer, think about how broad and complex our genetic structure is and how difficult it is to map at what point it has gone awry. And when researchers say that our cancers are as unique as our DNA, they mean that, while those of us with hormone-negative share many traits, we might have just as many elements that make us different.

Our DNA can repair itself when the system is working normally. And even when cancerous cells develop, the body can often deal with them by triggering programmed cell death (apoptosis) or by actions of the immune system. In fact, some critics say we overtreat cancer, diagnosing it before the body has had a chance to do its magic.

But this repair system does not always work because of genetic mutations. Researchers have found several genetic markers that are connected with hormone-negative breast cancer, especially basal-like tumors. These all could eventually lead to new hormone-negative treatment options. The most common are the BRCA genes, which are suspected in about half of all inherited breast cancers. Other markers are less common, such as the MAP gene. Tests on most of these markers are also less common, but I am presenting this information as a means of describing how hormone-negative cancer is different from others. And, perhaps, eventually we'll be regularly tested

BOX 4–3   **Genes and Basal-like Breast Cancers**

Basal-like breast cancers are usually triple-negative. They are also likely to be positive for cytokeratin 5/6 and EGFR, or Her1. They are strongly associated with mutations in the BRCA1, BRCA2, and p53 genes, and with the MAP gene.

Some researchers now talk about a whole new type of cancer—the five-negative subtype, which is triple-negative plus negative for cytokeratin 5/6 and EGFR, or Her1.

Nearly 15 percent of all breast cancers are basal-like, but 75 percent of all triple-negative cancers are basal-like. Basal-like cancers are likely to be diagnosed at later stages and with higher grades than other breast cancers, indicating that they grow rapidly, which may be why they come with a poorer prognosis.

is in the majority of breast cancers, but basal types have more of it.[5] Inhibitors already exist for this gene; scientists say that understanding this gene may lead to new treatment for triple-negative and other hormone-negative cancers.

Poly (ADP)-ribose polymerase (PARP): This pathway is another communication system the body uses to block the development of cancer cells. PARP helps a body repair its DNA. But cancer cells themselves use PARP, causing more DNA damage and making those cancer cells especially resistant to therapy. Researchers are analyzing how PARP inhibitors may interfere with the cancer cell's ability to repair its DNA. Used in conjunction with chemotherapy, these inhibitors may ultimately treat metastatic triple-negative, although research has shown mixed results of the inhibitors' effectiveness.

DEAR1 gene: This gene develops in the ducts of the breast and in the glands. Early research shows that women with triple-negative and a family history of breast cancer who express this gene may have a better prognosis than those without it.[6]

Aurora-A: This enzyme is important for healthy cell proliferation. Estrogen-negative tumors with high levels of it may be taxane-resistant.[7]

The Interplay of Hormones and Receptors

Hormones are necessary for the healthy functioning of our bodies, controlling our reproductive systems, brain, and other organs such as our thyroid, liver, and pancreas. In a healthy body, they function together like a well-run internal factory. When one hormone is off balance, though, it can affect the entire body.

Hormones are created in the endocrine system, which controls the body's growth and development, metabolism, and tissue function. Hormones are actually regulators, influencing the activity of cells and organs. Scientists call hormones "chemical messengers" because they deliver information from cell to cell; that information affects the way our bodies function. This communication works through receptors—cells can communicate only with other cells that have the appropriate receptors.

In hormone-negative breast cancer, cells cannot communicate successfully because of a lack of receptors. This is why tamoxifen and Arimidex and other hormone therapies don't work—they communicate with receptors to repair the cellular damage cancer causes. Without receptors, hormone-negative cells cannot get the message from these drugs to the cancer.

In women's bodies, estrogen and progesterone are complementary hormones. While we often focus on estrogen, it can function properly only in connection with progesterone.

Estrogen is produced primarily by the ovaries and, during pregnancy, the placenta; other sources of small amounts are the adrenal glands, liver, and breasts. In postmenopausal women, estrogen is produced by fat cells. It is responsible for the development of breasts and our ability to reproduce and also helps prevent bone loss. In pregnancy, it works with progesterone to prepare the lining of the uterus and nourish the developing fetus.

In cases of mixed receptor status—positive for estrogen and negative for progesterone, for example—estrogen is the primary determining factor in whether a tumor will respond to hormone therapy such as tamoxifen.[8] Estrogen-positive tumors respond, even those that are also progesterone-negative.

The major tenet of estrogen-negative breast cancer is that it is not fueled by estrogen. However, estrogen may be involved in the initial development of the disease. Estrogen-positive progenitor cells—the initial cells in cancer development—can cause nearby

TABLE 4–1   Progesterone and Breast Cancer[a]

In British research focused on the effects of progesterone, researchers determined that:

- ER+/PR– tumors had a better prognosis that ER-/PR-.
- ER–/PR+ tumors had essentially the same prognosis as ER-/PR-.
- ER+/PR- cancers were general smaller and had lower grades than ER–/PR– or ER–/PR+.

[a]Rakha, Emad A., El-Sayed, Maysa E., Green, Andrew R., Paish, E. Claire, Powe, Desmond G., Gee, Julia, Nicholson, Robert I., Lee, Andrew H. S., Robertson, John F. R., and Ellis, Ian O., "Biologic and clinical characteristics of breast cancer with single hormone receptor positive phenotype," *Journal of Clinical Oncology*, vol. 25, no. 30, 4772–4778 (2007), http://jco.ascopubs.org/content/25/30/4772.full.

estrogen-negative cells to grow, especially in cancers related to the BRCA mutation.[9] This may explain why young women are more likely to get triple-negative than older women.

Progesterone is produced by the ovaries, the adrenal gland, and, during pregnancy, the placenta. Working with estrogen, it helps regulate our menstrual cycles and sexual desire and prepares the body for childbirth. Premenstrual syndrome (PMS) may be the result of high levels of progesterone. Low levels may cause menstrual irregularities.

Progesterone's role in breast cancer has caused debate for years, with some researchers saying it has little effect, and others saying it is a significant predictor of recurrence. Women with estrogen-positive and progesterone-negative disease with no involved lymph nodes fared the worst in a study evaluating the separate effects of estrogen and progesterone on 1,944 British women and published in the *Journal of Clinical Oncology* (2007). For these women, the absence of progesterone alone was the only predictor of recurrence and shorter survival, regardless of tumor size, grade, or patient age.

Her2/neu, or the human epidermal growth factor receptor 2, is a protein that helps regulate normal cell growth. It is also called c-erbB-2. Like other receptors, it helps with signal transmission related to cell growth and differentiation. It is considered an onco-gene—a gene related to cancer. Cancers that are positive for Her2/neu are highly aggressive, but respond to the drug Herceptin. Triple-negative cancers are negative for her2/neu, in addition to being negative for estrogen and progesterone receptors. In most cases, it is a good thing to be negative for Her2 because it is such a highly aggressive receptor. The exception is when you are also negative for estrogen and progesterone receptors. The combination of the three—ER-negative, PR-negative and Her2-negative—creates a potent mix of negatives, again showing the complex set of interactions that build this disease.

Still, cancers that are Her2-positive can be more lethal than some harmone-negative breast cancers.

Epidermal growth factor receptor (EGFR): Also called Her1, EGFR belongs to a family of receptors that includes Her2, Her3, and Her4. It binds to cells and is part of a system that regulates cell growth and development. Some 60 percent of all basal-like breast cancers are positive for EGFR; cancers with EGFR are connected with an especially high rate of recurrence.[10,11] Inhibitors already exist for EGFR, including erlotinib (Tarceva), used to treat some lung and pancreatic cancers, and cetuximab (Erbitux), used for colorectal and head and neck cancers.

Insulin-like growth factor receptor 1 (IGF-1R): This receptor mediates the effects of the protein hormone IGF-1, which is similar in structure to insulin and may be overexpressed in many cases of triple-negative.[12]

Androgens are normally considered male hormones, the most common being testosterone. But they are also present in women's bodies, where they're produced in the ovaries, adrenal glands, and fat cells and ultimately are converted to estrogen. High levels of androgens are associated with both too much and too little hair, acne, infertility, and blood sugar disorders such as diabetes. Low levels are connected to fatigue, low libido, and a susceptibility to bone disease.

Now, scientists are studying the effect of androgens on triple-negative breast cancer. In research presented at the Impakt Breast Cancer Conference in Brussels, Belgium in 2009, patients who had triple-negative breast cancer and who also had androgen receptors tended to react less favorably to chemotherapy than those without the receptors.[13] A clinical trial is underway to study the role of androgen receptors in breast cancer.

Inflammation and the Insulin Connection

Inflammation is one of the body's responses to a weakened immune system. A weak system is often an inflamed one. Inflammation is implicated in a host of diseases—diabetes, arthritis, heart disease, digestive problems, and, of course, cancer. And triple-negative breast cancer has been associated in several studies with inflammation at the cellular level.[14,15] The inflammatory effect is usually nothing we can see or feel, but it is another biological difference between this and other cancers and may ultimately help researchers better understand this disease and how to treat it.

Metabolic syndrome is often correlated with inflammation and consists of a combination of risk factors such as high blood glucose, high blood pressure, and abdominal obesity, plus cholesterol problems like low HDL ("good" cholesterol), high LDL ("bad" cholesterol), and high triglycerides. Women diagnosed with triple negative breast cancer are much more likely to have metabolic syndrome than those with other forms of breast cancer.[16] Researchers at the Cleveland Clinic evaluated 176 patients, 86 who were triple negative and 90 who were not. Fifty-eight percent of triple negative patients had metabolic syndrome compared to only 36.7 percent of non-triple negative patients. Hypertension and a high body mass index (above 30) alone, however, were not associated with triple-negative.

In research using Women's Health Initiative data and published in the *Journal of the National Cancer Institute* (2011), low levels of exercise and a high body mass index were both risk factors for triple-negative. Of most significance was weight gain between the age of 35 and 50 and a body mass index above 31. Researchers analyzed records on 162,000 women, 3,116 of whom had complete tumor marker data; 307, or 10 percent, of these were triple-negative.[17]

Insulin resistance: According to the ongoing California Teachers Study (CTS), even though tumors of hormone-negative cancer do not need estrogen to grow, at the stem-cell stage they may be initially formed because of out-of-kilter hormones that are linked to insulin. So, while estrogen is not the perpetrator, it may be an accessory to the crime, aiding insulin in the initial formation of the disease.

The CTS collects health information from 133,479 current and former public school teachers or administrators who participate in the California State Teachers Retirement System. Research using these data has shown that moderate-to-strenuous exercise is a far more potent deterrent to hormone-negative cancer than it is to hormone-positive.[18] Insulin sensitivity might be why, because women who exercise are more likely to have lower levels of insulin in their blood and are more likely to maintain a normal body weight.

The Women's Intervention Nutrition Study (WINS) found similar connections to insulin and hormone-receptor-negative.[19] In that study, women with hormone-negative cancer benefited more from a low-fat diet than women with hormone-positive. Reducing dietary fat reduces insulin and insulin resistance. And while the WINS research focused on diet, some researchers say weight loss and exercise may be the real keys in reducing risk of recurrence, and both are related to insulin.

More evidence of the insulin influence comes from research in *The American Journal of Clinical Nutrition* (2008) showing that a diet heavy in simple carbohydrates—sugar, white bread, cakes and cookies—can put a woman at risk of hormone-negative breast cancer.[20] Researchers studied the diets of 62,739 postmenopausal women from 1993 to 2002; 1812 of these women eventually were diagnosed with breast cancer, 279 of those with estrogen-negative. Researchers found what they called a "direct association" between a high intake of simple carbs and estrogen-negative cancer. Because simple carbs are rapidly absorbed by the body, they note, they elevate insulin levels, which may be the link to hormone-receptor-negative breast cancer.

Research on the diabetes drug metformin also points to an insulin connection. Used in conjunction with Adriamycin, metformin effectively eliminated cancer stem cells in laboratory tests at the Harvard Medical School.[21] Researchers studied four genetically different cancer types, including triple negative, and determined that the drug combination eliminated existing tumors and prevented regrowth; neither drug alone was effective against the cancer cells. Clinical trials are being planned on the use of metformin and doxorubicin (Adriamycin) in women with early stage breast cancer.

None of these studies connects breast cancer and diabetes nor do they suggest that insulin sensitivity causes hormone-negative breast cancer. The basic message here is that everything in the body is connected in some way, and that an imbalance in one area can cause an eruption in another, with cancer as one possible—but not inevitable—result of this internal gurgling.

Reproductive Factors

One of the areas in which hormone-negative stands out as different from other types of breast cancers is, not surprisingly, in our reproductive histories. This area of study is evolving, but research has shown some surprising connections. The Life After Cancer Epidemiology (LACE) study offers one of the best in-depth views of the relationship between breast cancer and reproductive factors. Unless otherwise noted, the following information comes from LACE research.

Childbirth: Women with triple-negative, on average, had more children—at least three—than non-triple-negative women. And the more times a woman gave birth, the higher her risk of triple-negative breast cancer.

In fact, women who had never given birth had a 40 percent reduced risk of TNBC, according to Women's Health Initiative research published in the *Journal of the National Cancer Institute* (2011). They did face an increased risk of hormone-positive disease, however. Researchers speculated that this relationship may result from an abnormal response to pregnancy hormones.[22]

Breast feeding: Women with triple-negative breast cancer were less likely to breast-feed for more than four months and were more

---

BOX 4–4 Life After Cancer Epidemiology (LACE) Study

Researchers studied 2,280 women diagnosed with stage I, II, or IIIA breast cancer between 1997 and 2000. The women were 18 to 70 years old and 11 to 39 months postdiagnosis, free of recurrence.

11.3 percent were triple-negative
73.4 percent were luminal A
11.6 percent were luminal B
3.7   percent were Her2-positive

Source: Caan, Bette, Sternfeld, Barbara, Gunderson, Erica, Coates, Ashley, Quesenberry, Charles, and Slattery, Martha L., "Life After Cancer Epidemiology (LACE) Study: A cohort of early stage breast cancer survivors (United States)," Cancer Causes and Control, vol. 16, no. 5, 545–556 (2005).

likely to not breast-feed at all if they had at least three children. In African Americans, breast-feeding appeared to reduce the risk of TNBC for women who had multiple births.

Menstruation and menopause: Triple-negative women were younger at the onset of menstruation. If they were premenopausal, they were more likely to be overweight. Asians (59.1 percent) were less likely to be postmenopausal than Caucasians.

Hormone replacement therapy (HRT): Most studies tie HRT to hormone-positive but not to hormone-negative. In fact, according to research using California Teachers Study data and published in 2010, postmenopausal women who used HRT actually faced a slightly reduced risk of triple-negative; they did have an increased risk of hormone-positive.[23]

In the LACE study, luminal B and Her2-positive cases were the least likely group to have used hormone replacement therapy. And the great majority of Caucasians—76.2 percent—had used HRT.

Birth control: Women under the age of 40 who used oral contraceptives more than doubled their risk of triple-negative breast cancer.[24] There was no increase in the risk for hormone-positive breast cancer for oral contraceptive users.

How and Why Is Race a Risk Factor?

The fact that women of African ancestry tend to get hormone-negative breast cancer more frequently than other ethnic and racial groups is one of the most consistent patterns of this disease. This offers researchers some hope of defining specific risk factors for triple-negative as a whole. Several potential factors:[25]

Aneuploid tumors: African-Americans tend to have a higher incidence of this type of tumor, which is associated with chromosome abnormalities—too few or too many. This may indicate a form of breast cancer that is inheritable.

EZH2 stem cells: The protein EZH2 is expressed in a great majority (74 percent) of hormone-receptor-negative tumors, mostly triple-negative. It is linked to larger tumor size—more than 2 centimeters—and an increased likelihood of spreading to the lymph nodes.[26] Given that African Americans tend to have larger, more aggressive triple-negative tumors, there could be an

BOX 4–5   **Toxins in Our Environment**

Scientists agree that a wide variety of materials in our products, air, and work and home environments can put us at risk of cancer. No studies have specifically noted a connection to hormone-negative breast cancer, but in many cases, we can reduce our toxic dangers relatively easily, for an ounce of prevention.

Bisphenol A (BPA). Found in the lining of metal food cans and in plastic food containers, including some baby bottles, microwave ovenware, and eating utensils, BPAs have been connected to multiple types of cancer, but the research so far has focused on animals and not humans.[a] For example, in a 2010 study, mice exposed to BPAs in their mother's womb had an increased chance of cancerous tumors or of mammary gland changes in adulthood.[b] The study did not differentiate by receptor status.

Parabens. These chemicals are in cosmetics and personal care products such as lotions, makeup, and antiperspirants and have weak estrogen-like properties. Parabens have been found in breast cancer tumors, but whether or not they were responsible for the cancer is unclear.[c] Additional research is needed before we make any conclusions, but plenty of cosmetics are made without parabens, so why take a chance?

Phthalates. These plastic compounds are in baby powder, lotions, shampoo, and other personal care products. They are implicated in breast cancer because of their ability to disrupt the endocrine system, which balances hormonal development. In 2009 research in Northern Mexico, one specific type of phthalate, ethyl phthalate, was associated with breast cancer risk, but other phthalates showed no connection.[d] Phthalates can easily be avoided by buying chemical-free products.

For additional insight on breast cancer and the environment, check out the following:

- The Breast Cancer Fund, which "works to connect the dots between breast cancer and exposures to chemicals

(Continued)

BOX 4–5 (Continued)

and radiation in our everyday environments." For more information, go to the group's site at http://www.breastcancerfund.org.

- *Reducing Environmental Cancer Risk, What We Can Do Now*, 2008–2009 Annual Report, President's Cancer Panel. Download a free copy at http://deainfo.nci.nih.gov/advisory/pcp/annualReports/pcp08–09rpt/PCP_Report_08–09_508.pdf.
- *State of the Evidence: Breast Cancer and the Environment*, by Janet Gray, Ph.D., Janet Nudelman, M.A., and Connie Engel, Ph.D., which provides a thorough overview of the topic, looking at the effects of chemicals such as Bisphenol A (BPA), phthalates, parabens, pesticides, and herbicides. The authors include a section on how to act on current research. Download a free copy at http://www.breastcancerfund.org/assets/pdfs/publications/state-of-the-evidence-2010.pdf.
- The Breast Cancer and the Environment Research Centers, which consists of four cancer centers in the United States that are studying the effects of environmental factors on breast cancer risk. Included are the University of California at San Francisco, Michigan State Center, the University of Cincinnati Center, and the Fox Chase Cancer Center, plus numerous partnering institutions. The initiative is funded by the National Institute of Environmental Health Sciences and the National Cancer Institute. For more information on the Breast Cancer and the Environment Research Centers, go to the group's site at http://www.bcerc.org/new.htm.
- The Collaborative on Health and the Environment, a partnership of researchers, advocates, practitioners, and patients who are studying environmental risk on all forms of cancer. The group sponsors meetings, café calls, and online discussions. Check out the Collaborative on

BOX 4–5 **(Continued)**

Health and the Environment, and consider joining, at http://www.healthandenvironment.org/index.php.

[a]American Cancer Society, "Federal report looks at risks from plastics chemical," http://www.cancer.org/cancer/news/news/federal-report-looks-at-risks-from-plastics-chemical (accessed November 10, 2010).

[b]Doherty, Leo, Bromer, Jason G., Zhou, Yuping, Aldad, Tamir S., and Taylor., Hugh S., "In utero exposure to diethylstilbestrol (DES) or bisphenol-A (BPA) increases EZH2 expression in the mammary gland: an epigenetic mechanism linking endocrine disruptors to breast cancer," *Hormones and Cancer*, vol. 1, no. 3, 146–155 (2010).

[c]Darbre, P. D., Aljarrah, A., Miller, W. R., Coldham, N. G., Sauer, M. J., and Pope, G. S., "Concentrations of parabens in human breast tumours," *Journal of Applied Toxicology*, vol. 24, no. 1, 5–13 (2004).

[d]López-Carrillo, Lizbeth, Hernández-Ramírez, Raúl U., Calafat, Antonia M., Torres-Sánchez, Luisa, Galván-Portillo, Marcia, Needham, Larry L., Ruiz-Ramos, Rubén, and Cebrián, Mariano E., "Exposure to phthalates and breast cancer risk in northern Mexico," *Environmental Health Perspectives*, vol. 118, no. 4, 539–544 (2010).

association between EZH2 expression and tumors in women of African ancestry.

ALDH1: This genetic marker for breast cancer tissue is associated with an especially serious prognosis.[27] Women from Ghana are much more likely to have this marker than are white Americans or Europeans, suggesting this as a possible link to triple-negative.

Breast biology: It is possible that women of African descent simply have breast tissue that is more cancer-prone, making them more susceptible to aggressive cancer.

Men and Breast Cancer

Because men aren't typically known for their estrogen reserves, we might assume that the 1,500 or so men a year who get breast cancer would get hormone-negative. Research proves otherwise. In fact, in one study, 81 percent of breast cancers in men were estrogen-positive compared to about 75 percent for women.[28] Still, the odds are 100 to 1 against men getting breast cancer. Those who do are typically slightly older than women at diagnosis, with a median age of 68 compared to 63 for women. Curiously, the 100:1 ratio correlates with the approximate ratio of breast tissue in women and men, respectively.

African-American men, like African-American women, face a poorer prognosis than white men—they are three times more likely to die from breast cancer.[29] In addition, they are more likely than white men to have larger tumor sizes, cancer that has spread to the lymph nodes, more aggressive tumors, and higher rates of other illnesses.

As with women, hormonal abnormalities are a risk factor for men; these can be demonstrated by testicular problems such as undescended testes, congenital inguinal hernia, and testicular injury. Because 15 to 20 percent of men with breast cancer have a family history of the disease—compared to 7 percent of the general population—the researchers suspect that the BRCA1 and BRCA2 genes might be a factor in male breast cancer, so testing for these mutations is generally recommended for men diagnosed with breast cancer. Family history is a significant factor if other members were diagnosed before age 50. Other risk factors in men include infertility, Klinefelter syndrome (an extra "X" chromosome), benign breast conditions (nipple discharge, breast cysts, and breast trauma), radiation exposure, and Jewish ancestry. Jewish men most at risk are of Ashkenazi descent (Eastern European or Russian) with a family history of breast or ovarian cancer.

Nuts and Bolts

How to Use the Internet to Find Authoritative Information
The Internet is a treasure trove of excellent information. It is also a black hole of bad data and bad advice. The best sites inform and empower you; the worst scare your socks off. How do you tell the difference? Go with sites offered by established organizations. Some of the organizations and sites I have found especially helpful:

Triple Negative Breast Cancer Foundation (http://tnbcfoundation.org). With discussion forums, research updates, special events, and opportunities for involvement, this site is specifically for women with TNBC. The foundation also funds research on TNBC, with a goal being to "ignite interest in the study of triple negative breast cancer among researchers, physicians, educators, and scientists." With Living Beyond Breast Cancer, it cosponsors educational teleconferences on triple-negative. I occasionally guest blog for the foundation.

Living Beyond Breast Cancer (http://lbbc.org). Focused on what happens after treatment—how to "live as long as possible, with the best quality of life"—this group regularly sponsors telecasts on triple-negative, which are available as transcripts and podcasts afterward. In April, they sponsor an Ask-the-Expert session on triple-negative.

Facing Our Risk of Breast Cancer Empowered (FORCE) (http://www.facingourrisk.org). FORCE is a nonprofit organization for those with hereditary breast and ovarian cancer. It plans an annual conference and webinars on topics such as BRCA-associated breast cancer, and connects women to others in their community. The site includes research and information on cancer risk and risk management, a message board, opportunities for volunteering and fundraising, and advocacy options.

Breast Cancer.org (http://www.breastcancer.org). This site won the 2007 Platinum Award for Best Healthcare Content and the Silver Award for Best Overall Internet Site. It's full of great information to help you with everything from navigating your pathology report to understanding breast reconstruction. The group offers online Ask-the-Expert Conferences, chat rooms, and blogs. One conference, still available in the group's archives, dealt specifically with HR-disease. I am one of their guest bloggers.

Positives About Negative (http://hormonenegative.blogspot. com). This is my blog, which focuses on hormone-negative breast cancer, especially triple-negative.

American Cancer Society (http://www.cancer.org). Separate sections on the site are devoted to specific types of cancer, including breast cancer. The ACS offers a series of interactive tools that help you understand your treatment options, with pros and cons of different treatments, plus questions to ask your doctor. It also provides nutrition and exercise advice.

Dr. Susan Love Research Foundation (http://dslrf.org). This group's mission is to "eradicate breast cancer and improve the quality of women's health through innovative research, education and advocacy." The site is comprehensive, easy to navigate, and offers information that doesn't frighten, with an expert perspective and an engaging blog. Love, who is author *of Dr. Susan Love's Breast Book,* has a simple philosophy that is hard to beat: "We need to go beyond a cure. We need to stop people from ever getting breast cancer in the first place."

National Cancer Institute (http://cancer.gov). The Institute is part of the National Institutes of Health. The site has a special section on breast cancer, with statistics and details on research funded by the NCI and a breast cancer risk assessment interactive tool.

Susan G. Komen Breast Cancer Foundation (http:ww5//komen.org). Komen is probably the best-known breast cancer organization because of its Race for the Cure. The Komen site offers background information on breast cancer, news, and research reports, and it helps connect you to a support group. There's even an online breast exam.

UpToDate (http://www.uptodate.com). An online educational resource offering patients free access to current, in-depth patient information.

Photographic Profile

A Photographer Looks at Triple-Negative
Ever feel like a half-eaten apple? Open to your core, sort of left out to dry? Susan Landmann says that's what cancer did to her—made her feel exposed, damaged, bruised.

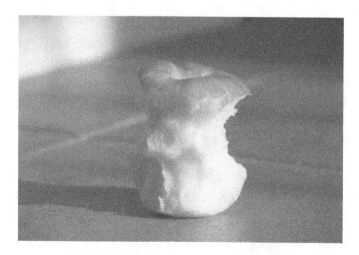

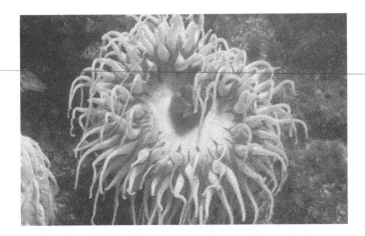

The apple analogy is especially apt because Susan was a teacher for 41 years until she fell off a desk while climbing to reach a bulletin board. (Ironically the board was intended to teach safety tips to her first-grade class.) She fractured her hip and pelvis, cracked the bone at the bottom of her spine, and tore off a bone in her knee. She couldn't walk for four months, and ended up retiring at the end of the year

"I'm sure that's what did in my immune system," she says. Susan was diagnosed with triple negative breast cancer less than a year after the fall, in August 2009, at 65. Before the fall, she had been a lifelong runner, hiker, and biker.

She is a photographer and she used her camera to help her explain how she felt throughout her diagnosis and treatment: Adriamcycln, Cytoxan, and Taxol. She did not tolerate any of the drugs well, ending up with joint pains, bloody noses, indigestion, fatigue, night sweats, peeling skin, and neuropathy. The ordeal threw her into depression.

One photo taken midway through shows the half-eaten apple: "This is how chemotherapy makes me feel," she says. Of another, featuring a sea anemone, she says, "This is how I imagine triple-negative might look."

After treatment, she continued regular walks through the moors by her Nantucket Island home and she started a rigorous low-fat, cancer-fighting diet. She talks with a therapist weekly. A year after diagnosis, she signed up for a course on photo essays in Maine. "School is tough," she says. "But I am loving it."[30]

Notes

1. http://www.myfightagainstbreastcancer.blogspot.com.
2. Molyneux, Gemma, Geyer, Felipe C., Magnay, Fiona-Ann A., McCarthy, Afshan, Kendrick, Howard, Natrajan, Rachael, Mackay, Alan, Grigoriadis, Anita, Tutt, Andrew, Ashworth, Alan, Reis-Filho, Jorge S., and Smalley, Matthew J., "BRCA1 basal-like breast cancers originate from luminal epithelial progenitors and not from basal stem cells," *Cell Stem Cell*, vol. 7, no. 3, 403–417 (2010).
3. Keam, Bhumsuk, Im, Seock A., Lee, Kyung H., Han, Sae W., Oh, Do Y., Kim, Jee H., Lee, Se H., Han, Wonshik, Kim, Dong W., Kim, Tae Y., Park, In A., Noh, Dong Y., Heo, Dae S., and Bang, Yung J., "Ki-67 can be used for further classification of triple negative breast cancer into two subtypes with different response and prognosis," *Breast Cancer Research*, vol. 13, no. 2, R22+ (2011).
4. Anders, Carey, and Carey, Lisa A., "Understanding and treating triple-negative breast cancer," *Oncology (Williston Park, N.Y.)*, vol. 22, no. 11 (2008). The Cancer Network has an accessible version of the research at http://www.cancernetwork.com/triple-negative-breast-cancer/content/article/10165/1340727.
5. Van Andel Research Institute, "Possible drug target found for one of the most aggressive breast cancers," news release, July 8, 2009, http://www.vai.org/News/News/2009/07_08_AggressiveBreastCancers.aspx (accessed October 22, 2010).
6. Lott, Steven T., Chen, Nanyue, Chandler, Dawn S., Yang, Qifeng, Wang, Luo, Rodriguez, Marivonne, Xie, Hongyan, Balasenthil, Seetharaman, Buchholz, Thomas A., Sahin, Aysegul A., Chaung, Katrina, Zhang, Baili, Olufemi, Shodimu-Emmanu, Chen, Jinyun, Adams, Henry, Band, Vimla, El-Naggar, Adel K., Frazier, Marsha L., Keyomarsi, Khandan, Hunt, Kelly K., Sen, Subrata, Haffty, Bruce, Hewitt, Stephen M., Krahe, Ralf Killary, and Ann M., "DEAR1 is a dominant regulator of acinar morphogenesis and an independent predictor of local recurrence-free survival in early-onset breast cancer," *PLoS Medicine*, vol. 6, no. 5, e1000068+ (2009). For a full copy of the article, go to http://www.plosmedicine.org/article/info%3Adoi%2F10.1371%2Fjournal.pmed.1000068
7. Bedard, Philippe L., Di Leo, Angelo, and Piccart-Gebhart, Martine J., "Taxanes: optimizing adjuvant chemotherapy for early-stage

breast cancer," *Nature Reviews Clinical Oncology*, vol. 7, no. 1, 22–36 (2009).

8. Pritchard, Kathleen I., "Tailored targeted therapy for all: a realistic and worthwhile objective against," *Breast Cancer Research*, vol. 11, Suppl. 3 (2009).

9. Wright, Mollie, Calcagno, Anna, Salcido, Crystal, Carlson, Marisa, Ambudkar, Suresh, and Varticovski, Lyuba, "BRCA1 breast tumors contain distinct CD44+/CD24- and CD133+ cells with cancer stem cell characteristics," *Breast Cancer Research*, vol. 10, no. 1, R10+ (2008).

10. Anders, Carey, and Carey, Lisa A., "Understanding and treating triple-negative breast cancer," *Oncology (Williston Park, N.Y.)*, vol. 22, no. 11 (2008). The Cancer Network has an accessible version of the research at http://www.cancernetwork.com/triple-negative-breast-cancer/content/article/10165/1340727.

11. Gonzalez-Angulo, Ana M., Litton, Jennifer K., Broglio, Kristine R., Meric-Bernstam, Funda, Rakkhit, Ronjay, Cardoso, Fatima, Peintinger, Florentia, Hanrahan, Emer O., Sahin, Aysegul, Guray, Merih, Larsimont, Denis, Feoli, Francesco, Stranzl, Heidi, Buchholz, Thomas A., Valero, Vicente, Theriault, Richard, Piccart-Gebhart, Martine, Ravdin, Peter M., Berry, Donald A., and Hortobagyi, Gabriel N., "High risk of recurrence for patients with breast cancer who have human epidermal growth factor receptor 2-positive, node-negative tumors 1 cm or smaller," *Journal of Clinical Oncology*, vol. 27, no. 34, 5700–5706 (2009).

12. Bhargava, Rohit, Beriwal, Sushil, McManus, Kim, and Dabbs, David J., "Insulin-like growth factor receptor-1 (IGF-1R) expression in normal breast, proliferative breast lesions, and breast carcinoma," *Applied Immunohistochemistry & Molecular Morphology*, vol. 19, no. 3, 218–225 (2011).

13. Loibl, Sibylle, "Androgen-receptor: a new drug target in breast cancer," IMPAKT Breast Cancer Conference, Brussels, Belgium (2009).

14. Marginean, Felicia, Rakha, Emad A., Ho, Bernard C., Ellis, Ian O., and Lee, Andrew H. S., "Histological features of medullary carcinoma and prognosis in triple-negative basal-like carcinomas of the breast," *Modern Pathology*, vol. 23, no. 10, 1357–1363 (2010).

15. Goodwin, Pamela, "Metabolic syndrome, insulin resistance, and inflammation in breast cancer: impact on prognosis and adjuvant interventions," *Current Breast Cancer Reports*, vol. 2, no. 4, 182–189 (2010).

16. Maiti, B., Kundranda, M. N., Spiro, T. P., and Daw, H. A., "The association of metabolic syndrome with triple-negative breast cancer," *Breast Cancer Research and Treatment*, vol. 121, no. 2, 479–483 (2010).

17. Phipps, Amanda I., Chlebowski, Rowan T., Prentice, Ross, McTiernan, Anne, Stefanick, Marcia L., Wactawski-Wende, Jean, Kuller, Lewis H., Adams-Campbell, Lucile L., Lane, Dorothy, Vitolins, Mara, Kabat, Geoffrey C., Rohan, Thomas E., and Li, Christopher I., "Body size, physical activity, and risk of triple-negative and estrogen receptor–positive breast cancer," *Cancer Epidemiology, Biomarkers and Prevention*, published first online March 1 (2011).

18. Find more information about the California Teachers Study at calteachersstudy.org/

19. Chlebowski, R. T., Blackburn, G. L., Thomson, C. A., Nixon, D. W., Shapiro, A., Hoy, M. K., Goodman, M. T., Giuliano, A. E., Karanja, N., McAndrew, P., Hudis, C., Butler, J., Merkel, D., Kristal, A., Caan, B., Michaelson, R., Vinciguerra, V., Del Prete, S., Winkler, M., Hall, R., Simon, M., Winters, B. L., and Elashoff, R. M., "Dietary fat reduction and breast cancer outcome: interim efficacy results from the Women's Intervention Nutrition Study," *Journal of the National Cancer Institute*, vol. 98, no. 24, 1767–1776 (2006).

20. Lajous, Martin, Boutron-Ruault, Marie-Christine, Fabre, Alban, Clavel-Chapelon, Francoise, and Romieu, Isabelle, "Carbohydrate intake, glycemic index, glycemic load, and risk of postmenopausal breast cancer in a prospective study of French women," *American Journal of Clinical Nutrition*, vol. 87, no. 5, 1384–1391 (2008). The full article is at http://www.ajcn.org/content/87/5/1384.full.pdf+html.

21. Hirsch, Heather A., Iliopoulos, Dimitrios, Tsichlis, Philip N., and Struhl, Kevin, "Metformin selectively targets cancer stem cells, and acts together with chemotherapy to block tumor growth and prolong remission," *Cancer Research*, vol. 69, no. 19, 7507–7511 (2009).

22. Phipps, Amanda I., Chlebowski, Rowan T., Prentice, Ross, McTiernan, Anne, Wactawski-Wende, Jean, Kuller, Lewis H., Adams-Campbell, Lucile L., Lane, Dorothy, Stefanick, Marcia L., Vitolins, Mara, Kabat, Geoffrey C., Rohan, Thomas E., and Li, Christopher I., "Reproductive history and oral contraceptive use in relation to risk of triple-negative breast cancer," *Journal of the National Cancer Institute*, vol. 103, no. 6, 470–477 (2011).

23. Saxena, Tanmai, Lee, Eunjung, Henderson, Katherine D., Clarke, Christina A., West, Dee, Marshall, Sarah F., Deapen, Dennis, Bernstein, Leslie, and Ursin, Giske, "Menopausal hormone therapy and subsequent risk of specific invasive breast cancer subtypes in the California Teachers Study," *Cancer Epidemiology, Biomarkers & Prevention*, vol. 19, no. 9, 2366–2378 (2010).The full article is at http://cebp.aacrjournals.org/content/early/2010/08/05/1055–9965.EPI-10–0162.full.pdf+html.

24. Dolle, Jessica M., Daling, Janet R., White, Emily, Brinton, Louise A., Doody, David R., Porter, Peggy L., and Malone, Kathleen E., "Risk factors for triple-negative breast cancer in women under the age of 45 years," *Cancer Epidemiology Biomarkers & Prevention*, vol. 18, no. 4, 1157–1166 (2009).

25. From a presentation by Lisa A. Newman, M.D., professor of surgery and director of the Breast Care Center at the University of Michigan, in a teleconference on triple-negative sponsored by Living Beyond Breast Cancer and the Triple Negative Foundation in April 2010.

26. Bandyopadhyay, S., Nahleh, Z., Ali Fehmi, R., Arabi, H., Sakr, W., Munkarah, A., and Kruger, M., "Enhancer of zeste homologue 2 (EZH-2) expression in breast cancer: a novel marker and potential target." American Society of Clinical Oncologists Annual Meeting, Orlando, Florida (2009).

27. Ginestier, Christophe, Hur, Min Hee H., Charafe-Jauffret, Emmanuelle, Monville, Florence, Dutcher, Julie, Brown, Marty, Jacquemier, Jocelyne, Viens, Patrice, Kleer, Celina G., Liu, Suling, Schott, Anne, Hayes, Dan, Birnbaum, Daniel, Wicha, Max S., and Dontu, Gabriela, "ALDH1 is a marker of normal and malignant human mammary stem cells and a predictor of poor clinical outcome," *Cell Stem Cell*, vol. 1, no. 5, 555–567 (2007).

28. Giordano, Sharon H., Buzdar, Aman U., and Hortobagyi, Gabriel N., "Breast cancer in men," *Annals of Internal Medicine*, vol. 137, no. 8, 678–687 (2002).

29. Crew, Katherine D., Neugut, Alfred I., Wang, Xiaoyan, Jacobson, Judith S., Grann, Victor R., Raptis, George, and Hershman, Dawn L., "Racial disparities in treatment and survival of male breast cancer," *Journal of Clinical Oncology*, vol. 25, no. 9, 1089–1098 (2007).

30. See more of Susan's work at http://susanlandmann.wordpress.com/.

5

Treatment: Your Options

A 4-CENTIMETER TUMOR TRANSLATES TO 1.5 INCHES, just slightly smaller than the diameter of a golf ball. By comparison, a 6-millimeter tumor is less than a quarter of an inch, smaller than a baby pea. These stats have real meaning to Sheri Nordstrom—before chemotherapy, her tumor was the golf-ball size; after, it had shrunk to pea size. And her two affected lymph nodes were cancer-free at the end of her six-month presurgery chemo regimen.

"It's on its way out," the pathologist said.

"Hooray for good chemo!" Sheri says.

Sheri, of Washington State, was diagnosed with triple-negative in 2005 at 37, when her first daughter was only three months old. She had a second daughter three years after treatment. And she is now more than six years past diagnosis.

Actually, she had found the lump about a month before her daughter was born, but dismissed it, thinking she was too young for breast cancer. Her doctor said it was most likely a clogged milk duct. "Let's wait and see," he said.

But the baby was born, her milk came in, and the tumor just kept getting larger. Finally, she had it tested and she got the bad news—triple-negative breast cancer. Her tumor had had the chance to grow and spread, and it warranted aggressive treatment.

Sheri had 12 rounds of Taxol weekly, then four rounds of dose-dense Adriamycin and Cytoxan. She then had a mastectomy on the affected breast—the right one—and removal of 12 lymph nodes, which were all negative at that point, followed by radiation. Several months later, after her sister was also diagnosed with breast cancer, she had her second breast removed.

She is BRCA-negative, but with a family history of cancer—one aunt with breast cancer, another with uterine, plus, now, her sister. A double mastectomy put her mind at rest. "I was paranoid, always waiting for the other shoe to drop," she says.

Chemo worked—she could feel the tumor shrink—but it also put her into temporary chemopause. She finished treatment in December 2005, and her periods resumed in February 2006. Nearly a year later, they stopped again, so she made an appointment with her ob-gyn. "What's up?" she asked. "Why am I not getting my period?" The doctor suggested a pregnancy test and, sure enough, she was pregnant—just weeks along.

"You must have the best doctor in the world," the obstetrician joked.

That pregnancy was uneventful, and her second daughter was born in October 2007, nearly two years after Sheri finished treatment, healthy and beautiful.

After chemo, she said, "I am not doing *that* again." Treatment was a trial, but it was successful, and five years later she is enjoying watching her two daughters grow. Her advice: "The road isn't always easy. There are days you want and need to cry. Give yourself a break sometimes—you don't always have to be the warrior, sometimes you need to be the patient. I encourage women to be their own advocate—know your treatment, know your options and if someone is doing something that doesn't seem right to you, seek a second opinion. And last but not least, never, ever give up hope."

Facing Treatment

My cancer was early stage, so my treatment was much less aggressive—a lumpectomy, four rounds of Adriamycin and Cytoxan, followed by six weeks of radiation. No taxanes. I had a small tumor and no affected lymph nodes. I still wonder if I needed chemotherapy, but

I am alive five years after the fact, with no signs of recurrence, so that is evidence that my treatment worked. Are my worsening arthritis and occasional memory lapses caused by chemo or the fact that I just turned 66? I will never know. I am a skeptic by nature, and would have loved to have been able to do an experiment on myself—one of me would take chemo, one would not. Given that I do not live in a *Star Trek* world, though, that's not likely to work. Research showing that chemotherapy is more effective against hormone-negative than against hormone-positive breast cancer, especially for those with no affected nodes, assures me a bit.

Still, because hormone-negative can come in such a broad range of forms, each woman's treatment should be tailored to her specific diagnosis. But deciding on that treatment can be stressful. You're reeling from a diagnosis and are still trying to come to grips with the fact that you, of all people, have cancer. And then you're told it is aggressive. You started out frightened, and the fear is building. In the midst of this, you have to make a decision that may save your life. Do you go for broke and choose the most aggressive treatment, or do you decide the risks are greater than the potential benefits?

Right now, treatment for hormone-negative typically consists of surgery, chemotherapy, and radiation. But new biologic agents intended to repair DNA damage specific to triple-negative are rapidly expanding the potential for treatment options.

Nuts and Bolts

Questions to Ask Your Doctor

Understanding your diagnosis is key to understanding your treatment. To decide the right path for you, use the questions below as the start of your discussion. Always ask how a treatment affects you specifically—if your doctor sounds like he is offering a cookie-cutter approach, it is time for a second opinion. No two women are the same; no two diseases are identical.

What clinical stage is my tumor? And what are the implications of that stage? See chapter 3 for more information on clinical stages.

What kind of surgery do you recommend and why? Why is that choice specifically better for me? If your surgeon recommends a mastectomy, ask for data that show that this approach is better for you than a lumpectomy. If, in contrast, you worry that a lumpectomy is enough, ask for data on its effects on your specific diagnosis.

Do I need chemotherapy? If so, should I have it before or after surgery? If I have it before, and the tumor responds to the chemo, what surgery would you plan afterward?

What is my prognosis with chemo? What is my prognosis without chemo? How will my individual risk be reduced? What is my individual risk of recurrence without chemo, and what is my risk of recurrence with chemo?

What chemo drugs do you use and why?

Do you have literature on those drugs, their effects, and their side effects? If he says, "We have taken care of the side effects," as one doctor told me, go elsewhere. They have not.

What type of radiation do you suggest? Is accelerated partial breast irradiation an option? What is its success potential in my specific case? Is whole breast radiation better? If so, why?

What about reconstruction? Will I need it? Do you recommend it? If so, should I have it done immediately or should I delay it until after treatment?

Can I talk to other women who have gone through this treatment? Hearing from actual women is good. This does not necessarily mean a support group—it means being able to call a smart woman who has already walked this road and talk with her about how that feels.

Surgery: Lumpectomy Versus Mastectomy

Surgery is usually a given for breast cancer of all types; options vary from the minimum to the maximum. In most instances it is the first step. In some cases, however—with large tumors or those that are difficult to reach—doctors may choose to do chemo first.

Lumpectomy: Also called a partial mastectomy, a lumpectomy takes only the cancerous portion of the breast, plus enough surrounding tissue to ensure removal of the entire tumor. Other terms for this operation include breast conservation surgery, quadrantectomy, segmental excision, wide excision, or tylectomy.

Lumpectomies can be done as outpatient surgery. I went to the hospital at 6 a.m. and was home by noon. I took one pain pill and was back at work the next day. I now wonder what the heck my hurry was, but this does demonstrate that the operation can be nothing to fear.

Doctors usually recommend lumpectomies for smaller (under 4 cm) tumors that are easily operable. It requires radiation afterward—five to seven weeks of daily treatment.

The most successful lumpectomies are those with *clear, or negative, margins*. This means that the cancer has not extended beyond the edge of the tissue taken. By comparison, *positive margins* means the cancer continues to the edge of the tissue. And with *close margins*, there is a minimal amount of cancerous tissue at the edges. Different hospitals define the amount of margins differently. My surgeon called mine clear, at a 0.3-centimeter distance to the closest edge.

If you have positive margins, doctors may do a second surgery and might suggest a mastectomy.

A lumpectomy with clear margins plus radiation is as successful in reducing risk of recurrence as a mastectomy for tumors under 4 centimeters, according to research in the *New England Journal of Medicine* (2002) that followed women 20 years after surgery.[1]

Mastectomy: A *simple mastectomy* removes the entire breast; a *radical mastectomy* removes the breast and the *axillary lymph nodes*, or the lymph nodes in the armpits. A *bilateral mastectomy*, or *double mastectomy*, removes both breasts. A *contralateral mastectomy* means removing the unaffected breast, or the breast opposite the affected, one—which is, of course, in addition to removing the affected breast. This is done to reduce chances of cancer on the opposite side.

Doctors use mastectomies for larger tumors (more than 4 cm). But the placement of even a small tumor may require a mastectomy—if, for example, it is far into the chest wall or if it is close to the nipple and surgery would be disfiguring.

A mastectomy is a far more extensive operation with greater risks and a longer recuperation time than a lumpectomy. Afterward, many women opt for breast reconstruction, although some are comfortable with no breasts—some even enjoy it. In her blog *Sex, Cancer, Etc.*, photographer Deborah Lattimore says, "I love my new body," and shows a photograph of herself with neat surgical lines where her breasts had been removed as part of her treatment for triple-negative.[2] She opted out of reconstruction.

Radiation is recommended after a mastectomy for those with large tumors or four or more affected lymph nodes.

I considered a mastectomy for peace of mind, but the research I did proved to me that, in my case, it was unnecessary. Having most of my body intact makes me feel more normal and helps me forget that I had breast cancer.

Surgical options are generally the same for hormone-negative as they are for hormone-positive with the same tumor characteristics. Recent studies, however, have shown some unique responses to surgery among specific subsets of triple-negative women patients.

• Women under 50 with stage I or II estrogen-negative breast cancer benefit the most from having a double mastectomy, although the benefit, researchers say, is small—a 4.8 percent reduced relative risk, according to a study published in the *Journal of the National Cancer Institute* (2010).[3]

BOX 5–1   **Relative Risk**

A reduced relative risk of 4.8 percent refers to the benefit in relation to your initial risk. That is, if your doctor says you have a 10 percent risk of recurrence, and a double mastectomy might reduce that risk by 4.8 percent, this means your risk is reduced by 4.8 percent of that original 10 percent, for a total reduced risk of less than a half percent. Relative risk can also be used to refer to risk in comparison to other groups, so the risk of breast cancer for women who have had babies might be compared with the risk of those who have not given birth.

The study used Surveillance Epidemiology and End Results (SEER) data on 107,106 women who underwent a mastectomy plus 8,902 who underwent a double mastectomy. Young women, who represented less than 10 percent of the group, benefited most. For women over 60, researchers found little benefit for a double mastectomy. However, they note, the research did not take into account factors such as the BRCA mutation or family history.

• Women with stage IV triple-negative breast cancer tumors are much less likely to benefit from surgery than those with hormone-positive or Her2-positive disease, according to a study at Memorial Sloan-Kettering Cancer Center in New York, published in the journal *Cancer* (2010). Researchers evaluated 186 patients with stage IV tumors, 68 of whom had surgery. Those with estrogen-positive, progesterone-positive, and Her2-negative saw improved survival rates with surgery. Those with triple-negative, however, had no survival benefit.[4]

• Extensive surgery can reduce the risk of developing a new breast cancer for women with the BRCA mutation. In an analysis of ten existing studies, an operation called *salpingo-oophorectomy*, or surgery to remove the ovaries and fallopian tubes, can reduce the risk of breast cancer by 50 percent in women with the BRCA1 or BRCA2 mutation.[5] Nevertheless, the researchers, writing in the *Journal of the National Cancer Institute* (2009), note that the surgery is not the only route to risk reduction. Mastectomy and regular MRI screenings have also been effective.

Lymph node dissection: The current standard for all forms of breast cancer is *sentinel node dissection* to determine if the cancer has spread to the lymph nodes. Immediately before surgery, doctors inject dye into the tumor and trace its route. It will go first to the sentinel node. The dye highlights the sentinel node, which is removed, along with one or two surrounding nodes, which are all tested for cancer. Instead of using dye, some cancer centers inject a radioactive tracer 12 hours before surgery; like dye, the tracer follows the path of the cancer. If the cancer has spread to the sentinel or other nodes, the patient will have a full *axillary lymph node dissection*, or removal of armpit nodes.

However, according to a phase III clinical trial published in *JAMA: The Journal of the American Medical Association* (2011), women with tumors smaller than 2 centimeters who were treated with lumpectomy, radiation therapy, and chemo did not benefit from having those additional lymph nodes removed. This was true no matter the hormone status of the tumor, so it would be true of triple-negative breast cancer. Researchers clarify that this does not apply to women who are at a high risk for recurrence such as those with three or more positive sentinel lymph nodes, larger tumors, or those who received preoperative chemotherapy. Five-year survival rates were 92.5 percent for those with no additional surgery and 91.8 percent for those with axillary lymph node dissection.

Doctors say this research may be a game changer, leading to fewer removals of the lymph nodes, a surgery that can lead to lymphedema, chronic pain, and limited range of motion.[6]

Chemotherapy and TNBC

Surgery is a local treatment—it takes care of a tumor in one location.

Chemotherapy is systemic—it targets the entire body, so it can kill local as well as distant cancer cells.

Chemo works by killing rapidly growing cells, which are usually cancer cells, but can also include cells in the hair, fingernails, skin, mouth, the lining of the stomach and intestines, and the bone marrow. It can target known tumors or fight possible micro-metastases doctors cannot even see yet.

It's this latter issue that causes some women concern: How do I know those micro-mets are out there at all? Am I fighting an existing disease, or am I putting my body through hell for something that might not even exist? We're targeting an unknown and unseen enemy; yet, we did develop the original tumor, so there is reason to believe that our bodies might contain more cancer.

Research can shine a light on what we cannot see, however. And research demonstrates that chemo is an effective line of defense against hormone-receptor negative breast cancers.

Chemotherapy can work in multiple ways: It can stop cancer cells from reproducing by altering the structure of the DNA of those cells; it can interfere with the creation of new cells, which blocks the formation of new DNA; or it can stop the mitotic process—the point at which a cancer cell divides into two cells.

Researchers think that, most of the time, the chemo does not kill all of the cancer cells. Some are resistant, dormant, or hiding in areas where tests cannot spot them. Those residual cells are either killed by the woman's immune system or eventually give rise to recurrent or metastatic disease, or both.

Before or After Surgery?

Why did I have chemo after surgery while Sheri had it beforehand? My tumor was smaller, so doctors felt they could get all the local cancer with surgery, then target any potential residual disease with chemo. In Sheri's case, chemo shrunk the tumor itself and the cancer that had spread to her lymph nodes, in addition to targeting any potential distant spread. This meant her surgical margins were much clearer because she had chemo beforehand.

Neoadjuvant chemotherapy is given before surgery. The word *adjuvant* means *furnishing additional support*. The prefix *neo* refers to modified. Doctors typically reserve neoadjuvant chemotherapy for cases in which surgery is difficult—with especially large tumors that mean major surgery; those that have spread, or metastasized, and would require multiple surgeries; or those that are difficult for a surgeon to safely or effectively reach.

In neoadjuvant therapy, the patient and medical team can see physical evidence of its effects—the tumor shrinks from one test to another. At surgery, the tissue that is removed can be carefully analyzed to get additional insight into how well the chemotherapy worked. In Sheri's case, an ultrasound and PET scan initially showed a 4-centimeter tumor; six months later, after neoadjuvant chemo, it was less than one-sixteenth that size.

With neoadjuvant therapy, the surgeon can then operate with less trauma to surrounding tissue and greater hope of removing any residual tumor cleanly. In some cases, it may be possible to avoid doing a mastectomy and do a lumpectomy instead. It also offers a real sense of how well that chemo regimen works in a particular woman because doctors can see how much the tumor shrinks.

The effectiveness of neoadjuvant chemotherapy is measured by how well the tumor has shrunk, or responded to the drugs, which can range from the tumor completely disappearing to the tumor not changing at all.

Complete pathological response: Women with triple-negative whose neoadjuvant therapy destroys the entire tumor have an especially good prognosis. This is called a complete pathological response (pCR), which means that all clinical evidence of the tumor is gone—there is no sign of the cancer after surgery. Sheri, for example, had a complete pathological response in terms of her lymph nodes—there was no sign of cancer after they were removed. Women with residual disease—some of the cancer remains—have a poorer prognosis, especially in the first three years.

In research in the *European Journal of Cancer* (2004), more than 75 percent of women with hormone-negative cancer who had neoadjuvant therapy saw their tumors shrink by more than half; 20 percent had a pathologically complete response.[7]

BOX 5–2   **TNBC Response to Neoadjuvant Chemotherapy**

Of 1,118 patients who received neoadjuvant chemotherapy at MD Anderson Cancer Center for stage I–III breast cancer from 1985 to 2004:

   255, or 23 percent, had TNBC.

   For patients with TNBC: 22 percent had a complete pathological response; three-year overall survival rates for these were 94 percent. For those without a complete pathological response, the three-year survival rate was 68 percent.

   For patients with hormone-positive: 11 percent had a complete pathological response; three-year overall survival rates for these were 98 percent. For those without a complete pathological response, the three-year survival rate was 88 percent.

Source: Liedtke, Cornelia, Mazouni, Chafika, Hess, Kenneth R., André, Fabrice, Tordai, Attila, Mejia, Jaime A., Symmans, W. Fraser, Gonzalez-Angulo, Ana M., Hennessy, Bryan, Green, Marjorie, Cristofanilli, Massimo, Hortobagyi, Gabriel N., and Pusztai, Lajos, "Response to neoadjuvant therapy and long-term survival in patients with triple-negative breast cancer," *Journal of Clinical Oncology*, vol. 26, no. 8, 1275–1281 (2008), http://jco.ascopubs.org/content/26/8/1275.full.

Partial response: Some disease remains in the body, but it has decreased by 30 percent or more in size or number of lesions. While less positive than a complete response, partial response nevertheless shows that chemo has worked. Sheri had a partial response.

Stable disease: The disease has a small or no decrease in size and number of lesions. A decrease of less than 30 percent or a slight increase in size is generally considered stable disease.

Progressive disease: A 20 percent increase in the size of lesions or the appearance of new lesions.

Adjuvant chemotherapy: This refers to chemo after surgery. Without the prefix *neo*, it simply means *providing support.* That is, it supports surgery. Smaller, localized tumors like mine—under 4 centimeters with minimal affected lymph nodes—are usually treated with surgery first, followed by adjuvant chemotherapy The surgery can effectively get rid of the cancerous tumor, and chemo kills whatever cancer cells might remain, but that the doctors can't see.

Dosage

As patients, our eyes may glaze over when doctors begin talking about dosage levels of chemotherapy—there's so much to learn, to absorb. I, for one, was not a good healthcare consumer in this regard. It was only months after treatment that I learned that the dose-dense regimen I got was actually good news. If your physician suggests using a less aggressive or "milder" chemotherapy, seek another opinion.

Dose-dense chemotherapy (DDC): This has become the standard and means chemo every two weeks. The theory is that chemo treatments packed closer together have more of a chance to kill cancer cells early, reducing their ability to divide and grow between treatments. This is especially important in fast-growing cancers such as hormone-negative, Her2-positive, and those in women under 50; DDC has been most effective in treating those groups.[8] It also allows you to get through chemo faster, somewhat reducing the disruption in your life.

Doctors in the past had been more conservative, giving patients three weeks between doses to rebuild their white blood counts. With the advent of drugs like Neupogen, Neulasta, and Leukine, which rebuild white blood cells, this is less of an issue.

But, while these drugs work well, they can add significantly to the already enormous costs of chemo—one injection can cost thousands of dollars. Check with your doctor first, to make sure your insurance covers the drug, or see if you can get any financial support for the treatment. Neupogen can cost a little less than Neulasta. My oncology team never mentioned cost to me when they scheduled Neulasta—they did note several times that it was "that drug you see advertised on TV." I had excellent insurance, so I guess they figured I was covered, so why worry. I was stunned to see how much they had billed my insurance company—more than $3,000 a shot. I have read recently of charges for the drug reaching $9,000.

High-dose chemotherapy (HDCT): This is an even more aggressive treatment and can destroy bone marrow along with cancer cells, which usually necessitates aggressive follow-up treatment such as a bone marrow transplant. Recent studies have shown that HDCT might be effective against triple-negative, but it remains experimental, with the need for much more research, specifically clinical trials.[9]

Weekly dosage: In some aggressive cancers, doctors combine chemotherapy drugs and give them weekly before surgery. Taxanes are often given weekly.

Nuts and Bolts

The Decision
The final choice of treatment is yours. Your doctor will provide options and will make recommendations. But for this to work, you need to be on board. Understanding what is possible and why makes your decision easier. To help you process, here's an overview of some options for hormone-receptor negative breast cancer:

Lumpectomy:
- For tumors under 4 centimeters
- Less invasive surgery, usually outpatient
- Requires radiation afterward
- Clear margins indicate all signs of the tumor were removed

- Positive or close margins may require more surgery
- Lumpectomy plus radiation is as effective as mastectomy

Mastectomy

- For larger (more than 4 cm) or difficult-to-operate tumors
- Extensive surgery with longer recuperation time
- Many women follow with reconstruction; many don't
- A double mastectomy can be most beneficial for women under 50
- Followed by radiation in the case of large tumors or those with four or more affected lymph nodes

Adjuvant Chemotherapy

- Done after surgery
- For tumors under 4 cm, especially those with minimal local spread
- More successful in fighting early stage hormone-negative than hormone-positive

Neoadjuvant Chemotherapy

- Done before surgery
- For tumors larger than 4 cm, especially with distant metastases, multiple local tumors, or multiple affected lymph nodes
- May also be used for difficult-to-reach tumors
- Pathologically complete response afterward offers a highly positive prognosis

Radiation

- Standard after a lumpectomy
- Generally involves radiation to the entire breast with a "boost" to the tumor
- May include radiation to the axillary nodes
- Used after a mastectomy in cases of tumors larger than 5 cm and four or more affected lymph nodes
- External beam radiation irradiates tumor site and surrounding breast tissue and is the commonest technique used
- Accelerated partial breast irradiation (APBI) involves a short course of radiation given just to the lumpectomy site
- Brachytherapy is one form of APBI. It uses radiated beads placed in the tumor site or in a balloon catheter, leaving the rest of the breast unaffected; must be done soon after surgery

Chemotherapy Drugs

The most common treatment for triple-negative combines Adriamycin, Cytoxan, and a taxane, although some centers now use a Cytoxan-taxane combination without the Adriamycin. Newer chemo drugs are being tested for triple-negative breast cancer, especially for locally advanced (node-positive or more than one tumor) and metastatic breast cancer.

All have side effects, some of which I list below; ask for detailed information from your doctor on all side effects, common and uncommon. Some patients experience few side effects, other are seriously incapacitated, and most are in between. These are serious drugs; they are essentially poisons that target cancer, but affect much of the rest of the body in the process.

Different women react to chemotherapy differently. In general, it's best to get started as soon as you can to avoid unnecessary worry and to kill the cancer ASAP. You could be one of the lucky women who face only limited side effects.

Anthracyclines and Alkylating Agents

These drugs prevent cancer cell division by disrupting the structure of the DNA.

Box 5–3   First-Line Versus Second-Line Drugs

First-line drugs are those that are commonly used on initial diagnosis, especially for disease that has not spread beyond the lymph nodes. This includes taxanes, alkylating agents such as Cytoxan and anthracyclines such as Adriamycin.

Second-line drugs are used when a tumor recurs, fails to respond to first-line drugs, or in especially aggressive cases. These include antimetabolites such as Xeloda, platinum agents such as cisplatin, and microtubule inhibitors such as Ixempra.

Doxorubicin

Brand Name: Adriamycin

Used For: Breast cancer as well as cancer of the bladder, head and neck, liver, lung, lymphomas, ovary, pancreas, prostate, stomach, thyroid, uterus, plus some types of leukemia and lymphomas. Developed in the 1950s from soil samples from Italy and France, it is now created chemically.

Possible Side Effects: An anthracycline, Adriamycin can cause damage to the heart muscle, especially when given for long periods of time, so doctors give patients a MUGA (multiple-gated acquisition) scan beforehand to make sure their hearts can handle the stress of the drug. This test demonstrates the strength of the heart's major pumping chamber, the left ventricle.

Other side effects include hair loss, a decrease in white blood cells, nausea, vomiting, constipation, and mouth sores; less common are skin eruptions on the palms of the hand or soles of the feet, swelling, pain, and erythema, or redness of the skin. Adriamycin can also interfere with fertility, causing periods to cease, in some cases temporarily, in others permanently. It slightly increases a patient's risk of leukemia.

Cyclophosphamide

Brand Name: Cytoxan

Used For: Breast cancer plus leukemia and ovarian cancer. It is derived from the infamous mustard gas used in World War I.

Possible Side Effects: An alkylating agent, Cytoxan suppresses production of white blood cells, red blood cells, and platelets, reducing the ability of the body to fight infection, impairing the blood's ability to clot blood, and reducing oxygen in the blood. Side effects include hair loss, vomiting, nausea, constipation, poor appetite, and sterility. Less common are mouth sores, diarrhea, and bladder irritations. Cytoxan also may affect the heart and lungs. Some patients have an increased risk of blood cancers such as leukemia.

EPIRUBICIN

Brand Name: Ellence in the United States; in other countries it is called Pharmorubicin or Epirubicin Ebewe.

Used For: Doctors may prescribe epirubicin, an anthracycline, because it has fewer side effects than Adriamycin. It is a relatively new drug, developed in the 1980s and approved by the FDA only in 1999, so it does not have the track record of Adriamycin. It was approved in Europe in the mid-1980s and is mostly used for patients whose cancers have spread to the lymph nodes.

Possible Side Effects: Nausea, hair loss, mouth sores, diarrhea, low energy, hot flashes, loss of appetite, and changes in menstrual periods.

Platinum Agents

Newly developed as therapy for cancer treatment, these drugs attack the DNA of cancer cells, creating a platinum complex inside the cancer cell that ultimately kills it.

CARBOPLATIN

Brand name: Paraplatin

Used For: Metastatic ovarian cancer. Research is under way to test its use for women with metastatic triple-negative breast cancer.

Possible Side Effects: Nausea and vomiting, hair loss, weakness, changes in taste, low red and white blood cells and platelets. Less common are abdominal pain, diarrhea, constipation, mouth sores, neuropathy (nerve damage), and hearing loss. Carboplatin is a newer platinum agents, and it may be less toxic in comparison to cisplatin, especially having fewer kidney-related side effects.

CISPLATIN

Brand name: Platinol-AQ and Platinu

Used For: Testicular, ovarian, or bladder cancers. Cisplatin is an old drug—first introduced in the 1800s for a variety of cancers—but scientists are just recently refining and testing its use for triple-negative breast cancer.

Possible Side Effects: Nausea and vomiting, kidney problems, and low white and red blood counts. Less common are hair loss, loss of appetite, changes in taste, especially a metallic taste, neuropathy (nerve damage), and changes in fertility.

Antimetabolites

These drugs include some of our oldest chemotherapeutic agents. They kill cancer by interfering with its metabolic process.

Fluorouracil (5-FU)

Brand Name: Adrucil, Carac, Efudex, and Fluoroplex

Used For: This drug was once a mainstay of chemotherapy, but now is seldom used for breast cancer in the United States, although it is still used elsewhere. In addition to breast cancer, it can be used for colon, rectal, gastrointestinal, head and neck, liver, and ovarian cancers. It is available as a topical cream for basal cell skin cancer.

Possible Side Effects: Low blood counts, diarrhea, mouth sores, changes in taste, and poor appetite. Less common are nail changes, darkening of the skin, and hair thinning.

Capecitabine

Brand name: Xeloda

Used For: Metastatic breast cancer that has not responded to paclitaxel and an anthracycline-containing chemotherapy regimen. Also used for stage III breast cancer and colon and colorectal cancer.

Possible Side Effects: diarrhea, nausea, vomiting, abdominal pain, fatigue, and weakness. More serious side effects include fever, chest pain, numbness, and slow heart rate.

Microtubule Inhibitors

Microtubules are essential elements in cell division. Microtubule inhibitors kill cancer by disrupting this process, essentially disrupting cancer's cellular balance.

IXABEPILONE

Brand Name: Ixempra

Used For: Primarily for metastatic or node-positive breast cancer that is resistant to treatment with more common drugs such as anthracyclines and taxanes.

Possible Side Effects: Headache, hair loss, weakened nails, mouth sores, loss of appetite, weight loss, nausea, vomiting, diarrhea, constipation, muscle and bone pain, tiredness, and difficulty tasting food. More serious effects include fever, dizziness, and hives.

Taxanes

These are both microtubule inhibitors and antimitotic agents that stop cancer cell division. Originally derived from the yew tree, the original taxane, paclitaxel, became the center of an environmental controversy in the 1970s and 1980s because its production used the Pacific yew tree and furthered the destruction of the world's old growth forests. The drug's production was ultimately modified, and it is now created chemically, from cultured cells.

PACLITAXEL

Brand Name: Taxol, Abraxane, and Apo-Paclitaxel in the United States; Aclixel, Asotax, Bristaxol, Cryoxet, Praxel, and Taxol Konzentrat elsewhere.

Used For: Node-positive breast cancers or those with large tumors. Also used for ovarian and lung cancers and for Kaposi sarcoma.

Possible Side Effects: Low white and red blood counts, nausea, diarrhea, mouth sores, hair loss, fatigue, weakness, weight gain, fluid retention, numbness in the fingers and toes, nail changes, vomiting, sterility, swelling of the ankles, shortness of breath, and low platelet count. Less common are muscle and bone pain and low platelet count. Some effects of the drug might not occur until years after treatment.

DOCETAXEL

Brand Name: Taxotere

Used For: Node-positive breast cancers or those with large tumors. Also used for lung, head and neck, gastrointestinal, and prostate cancers. Research shows that fewer doses of docetaxel can be as effective as more frequent doses of paclitaxel. In a 2008 clinical trial, patients with docetaxel as adjuvant therapy every three weeks did as well as those with weekly paclitaxel.[10]

Possible Side Effects: Low white and red blood counts, nausea, diarrhea, mouth sores, hair loss, fatigue, weakness, weight gain, fluid retention, numbness in the fingers and toes, nail changes, vomiting, sterility, swelling of the ankles, shortness of breath, and low platelet count. Less common are muscle and bone pain and low platelet count. Some effects of the drug might not occur until years after treatment. Those taking docetaxel plus Cytoxan are at a slightly increased risk of acute myeloid leukemia.

NAB-PACLITAXEL

Brand Name: Abraxane

Used For: Advanced or metastatic breast cancers that have not responded to other cancer drugs. Also used to treat pancreatic, lung, and bladder cancer.

Possible Side Effects: Low white and red blood counts, nausea, diarrhea, mouth sores, hair loss, fatigue, weakness, weight gain, fluid retention, numbness in the fingers and toes, nail changes, vomiting, sterility, swelling of the ankles, shortness of breath, and low platelet count. Less common are muscle and bone pain and low platelet count. Some effects of the drug might not occur until years after treatment.

BOX 5–4 **Who Benefits from Taxanes?**

A review of 21 trials affecting nearly 36,000 women with early-stage breast cancer evaluated the benefits of adjuvant chemotherapy—after surgery—using taxanes versus those not using taxanes. Published in *Nature Reviews Clinical Oncology* (2009),[a] the analysis found:

- Taxanes provide a 5 percent improvement in disease-free survival and a 3 percent improvement in overall survival regardless of the type of taxane, its schedule of administration, lymph node involvement, or hormone-receptor status. Researchers call this a "modest improvement."
- Women under 50 with and without affected lymph nodes benefit from taxanes. Relative risk of recurrence for node-negative disease in this group was reduced by 36 percent; relative risk of recurrence for node-positive disease was reduced by 37 percent.
- Women 50–69 have less of a benefit—a 23 percent reduced relative risk of recurrence for node-negative and 17 percent for node-positive.
- Hormone-receptor status does not affect the benefit significantly for women under 50. Those with estrogen-negative cancers faced a relative risk reduction of 39 percent, and those with ER-positive had a 44 percent relative risk of reduction.
- In women 50–69, taxanes may provide less of a benefit to women with estrogen-positive (16 percent relative risk reduction) than estrogen-negative (33 relative percent risk reduction).
- For women under 50, the relative risk of recurrence after two years remains similar to the risk after 15 years. For women 50–69, however, the risk reduction occurs in the first two years, with little or no effect after that. This may be related to estrogen-receptor status, as women with ER-negative typically face the highest risk of recurrence within two years, while those with ER-positive disease face a sustained risk—over a longer period.

- Paclitaxel at 80 mg/m2 once a week or docetaxel at 100 mg/m2 every three weeks is superior to paclitaxel at 175 mg/m2 every three weeks following four cycles of AC.
- Doxorubicin and paclitaxel followed by once-weekly paclitaxel is more effective than standard AC with paclitaxel every three weeks.
- Improvements in the pathologically complete response rate do not always translate to improvements in disease-free survival or overall survival.
- ER status or Her2 status alone isn't a significant predictor of who will benefit from taxanes.
- Genetic factors that are still being studied may provide the most information on who benefits from taxanes. For example, tumors with the P-glycoprotein may be taxane-resistant, as are those with β-tubulin mutations. Tumors with the TP53 mutation, however, may be more sensitive to taxanes. But ER-negative tumors with high levels of Aurora-A may be taxane-resistant.

[a]Bedard, Philippe L., Di Leo, Angelo, and Piccart-Gebhart, Martine J., "Taxanes: optimizing adjuvant chemotherapy for early-stage breast cancer," *Nature Reviews Clinical Oncology*, vol. 7, no. 1, 22–36 (2009).

Biologic Therapies

As we saw in chapter 4, hormone-negative breast cancer is a biologically unique disease; biologic agents zero in on that uniqueness to target specific markers. These agents are paired with chemo drugs to create a chemobiologic treatment, which is used most often in metastatic breast cancer—cancer that has spread beyond the breast. Biological therapies that have been tested for hormone-negative breast cancer include VEGF and EGFR inhibitors.

VEGF and EGFR Inhibitors

VEGF inhibitor: A drug that starves the cancerous tumor by compromising its supply of blood, oxygen, and other nutrients. It binds to the *vascular endothelial growth factor (VEGF)*, a protein that stimulates the development and growth of blood vessels. Drugs that target the blood supply are also called antiangiogenic drugs.

BEVACIZUMAB

Brand Name: Avastin

Used For: Metastatic breast cancers in conjunction with chemo drugs. Avastin has been effective in fighting basal-like and other triple-negative cancers, but less successful in early breast cancer or other metastatic breast cancers. It is also used for brain, colon, kidney, and lung cancers.

In 2011 the FDA rescinded its approval of the drug for breast cancer. Critics said its costs—some $8,000 a month at that time— far outweighed its benefits. Its potential for success with metastatic triple-negative does not appear to have swayed the FDA.

The European Union, however, sees more benefit to the drug—or is less swayed by costs. The European Medicines Agency has taken the position that the benefits of Avastin plus Taxol outweigh the risks; it remains a recommended drug in the EU. Research continues on using the benefits of the drug, including it as part of neoadjuvant chemotherapy—before surgery.[11,12] Consistently, the drug has shown more benefit for women with triple-negative breast cancers than for hormone-positive breast cancers. And because there are fewer women with TNBC in the test groups, it can look like the drug's benefits are minimal. Let's hope the FDA will eventually be swayed by continuing research on the use of Avastin for triple-negative breast cancer, both early stage and metastatic.

Side Effects: Diarrhea, stomach pain, loss of appetite, dry mouth, increased thirst, dizziness, and hair loss. Less common are fever, swelling or rapid weight gain, numbness, headache, shortness of breath, and a slightly increased risk of bleeding and bowel perforation. It can worsen coronary artery disease or peripheral artery disease.

SORAFENIB

Brand Name: Nexavar

Used For: Provided in tablet form for renal cell and liver cancer; being tested for triple-negative breast cancer.

Side Effects: Rash and other skin problems, diarrhea, fatigue. Less common are high blood pressure, hair thinning, low white blood count, and poor appetite.

EGFR inhibitors: Drugs that interfere with the epidermal growth factor receptor. Also called Her1, this receptor is present in 60 percent of all basal-like tumors, making EGFR inhibitors a potentially powerful targeted therapy.

Erlotinib, Cetuximab, and Panitumumab

Brand Names: Tarceva, Erbitux, and Vectibix

Used For: In conjunction with chemotherapy for locally advanced or metastatic cancers of the breast, colon, pancreas, and lung.

Side Effects: Headache, diarrhea, nausea, cough, abdominal pain, fatigue, and skin rashes.

Radiation

Radiation is usually the final step in breast cancer treatment. Generally speaking, all women who are treated by lumpectomy should have radiation therapy to decrease the risk of recurrence. It is a local treatment, using high-energy radiation to kill the cancer cells in the area that is irradiated. Radiation therapy for breast cancer is divided into whole breast radiation (a treatment in which the entire breast is radiated) and accelerated partial breast radiation (APR; in which radiation is delivered to the lumpectomy cavity and surrounding tissues).

External beam radiation, the most common form of breast radiation, uses X-rays directly aimed at the tumor and nearby tissue. It is usually given five days a week for six weeks and most commonly treats the whole breast (or chest wall after mastectomy). It may also be used to treat the affected lymph nodes.

Accelerated partial breast radiation includes brachytherapy, intraoperative radiation therapy, and focused external beam radiation techniques. The important distinction is that the radiation is delivered just to the lumpectomy site after the tumor is removed, and that the course of treatment is shorter.

Brachytherapy uses radiated beads implanted in the tumor site or placed through a special balloon catheter. If it proves to be as effective as whole beam radiation, it can be an appealing choice, reducing treatment time from six weeks to one, and meaning less invasive treatment, saving most of the breast from radiation. It is generally done during the early postoperative period.

Its use for high-risk women, such as younger women with triple-negative, is controversial, however. These techniques are mostly used now for women at relatively low risk of local recurrence, such as older women with clear margins.

Intraoperative radiotherapy involves delivering a single high dose of radiation directly into the open surgical cavity at the time of lumpectomy.

Radiation is standard treatment after a lumpectomy to decrease the risk of local recurrence at the lumpectomy site. In fact, for most women, the success of lumpectomies is tied to radiation treatment afterward. Researchers believe than some women might be able to forgo radiation after a lumpectomy; at present, however, they're not clear on how to identify those women.

Doctors will also use radiation after a mastectomy in advanced cases of breast cancer, such as with bigger tumors (usually larger than 5 cm), four or more affected lymph nodes (or as few as one for premenopausal women), and with positive margins after surgery.

Tamoxifen and Arimidex

Neither of these drugs is recommended for women with hormone-receptor-negative breast cancer. Their use is called hormone therapy or endocrine therapy because it interferes with the action or development of estrogen, which is part of the endocrine system. Tumors that are negative for both estrogen and progesterone receptors have less than a 5 percent chance of responding to these drugs. In cases of mixed hormone receptor status—that is, negative for either estrogen or progesterone receptors and positive for the other—the role of the estrogen receptor is the most important predictor, so even if you are negative for estrogen receptors and positive for progesterone receptors, you likely will not respond to endocrine therapy.[13]

In fact, taking tamoxifen might increase a woman's risk of estrogen-negative breast cancer. Women who took tamoxifen for at least five years had more than a fourfold increased risk of estrogen-receptor-negative cancer in the second breast compared to women who were not treated with hormone therapy, according to research published in *Cancer Research* (2009). The drug reduced the incidence of estrogen-receptor-positive breast cancer by 60 percent, however. Keep in mind that it was only one study, and a small one at that—367 women with estrogen-receptor-positive cancer that had also spread to the second breast and a comparison group of 728 women with only a primary cancer.[14]

Tamoxifen is the generic name for the drug sold as Nolvadex, Istubal, and Valodex. It is an estrogen antagonist, a drug that blocks the effects of estrogen and is given most often to premenopausal women with hormone-positive breast cancer. Side effects are a possibility of blood clots, strokes, cataracts, and uterine cancer. Less severe are weight gain, vaginal dryness, leg cramps, hot flashes, and joint pain.

Arimidex is the brand name for the drug anastrozole, an aromatase inhibitor—that is, a drug that lowers the level of estrogen in the body. It is often given to postmenopausal women with hormone-positive disease. Side effects include bone pain, anxiety, depression, diarrhea, headache, hot flashes, and weight gain. It can worsen osteoporosis.

Herceptin

This drug treats Her2-positive breast cancers and is used in addition to chemotherapy drugs for those who are negative for estrogen receptors.

Herceptin is the brand name of the trastuzumab, a monoclonal antibody that slows or stops the growth of cells that overexpress—create too much—Her2/neu. It is given by injection. When taken along with chemotherapy, it can cause anemia and is linked to mild upper respiratory infections. When taken without chemo, side effects can include fever, chills, weakness, nausea, vomiting, diarrhea, head-aches, difficulty breathing, and rashes.

Herceptin may actually turn estrogen-receptor-negative sta-tus into positive, according to a study presented at the Endocrine Society annual meeting (2009). It's a two-step process, though, and the research was done on laboratory cells, not on human subjects. Still, it could ultimately provide much-needed therapy for hormone-receptor negative breast cancer, including triple-negative.

In the research, cells that were estrogen-receptor negative and Her2-positive were treated with trastuzumab (Herceptin); after 72 hours they were treated with the hormones estradiol and androstenedione. After that they were given aromatase inhibitors and antiestrogens. The tumors then reacted in much the way hormone-receptor-positive tumors do to aromatase inhibitors and antiestrogens.[15]

Combined Therapy for Hormone-Negative

Some of the most regular prescribed regimens for treatment of hor-mone-negative breast cancer are:

AC: Adriamycin and Cytoxan. This had once been the gold stan-dard for node-negative breast cancers that had not spread to the lymph nodes. This is the therapy I had—four treatments every two weeks of Adriamycin and Cytoxan. Some cancer centers are replacing it with therapies that replace Adriamcycin with a taxane.

TC: A taxane plus an alkylating agent, usually Cytoxan, which can be less toxic than Adriamycin. This is becoming more com-mon for node-negative breast cancer than AC.

ACT: Andriamycin and Cytoxan are given first, followed by a taxane, usually paclitaxel or docetaxel. It is used for node-posi-tive or metastatic breast cancer.

TAC: Adriamycin and Cytoxan, or another combination of an anthracycline and an alkylating agent, plus a taxane adminis-tered concurrently. This is usually for aggressive breast can-cers—large, locally advanced, or metastatic.

PET: An anthracycline, a taxane, and a platinum agent. Common regimens include Cisplatin, Epirubicin, and Paclitaxel. This is used for node-positive or metastatic breast cancer.

CMF: A combination of Cytoxan, methotrexate (Amethopterin, Mexate, Folex), and fluorouracil (5FU). This was one of the earliest drug regimens, which is being replaced by more modern treatments, but may still be used for women who cannot tolerate newer chemo drugs. Treatment schedules vary, but one approach is to give the drugs on the first day of treatment, with a second dose eight days later and a third three weeks after that, for one full cycle. Each cycle is repeated six to eight times.

Which Regimen Works Best?

The characteristics of your cancer as described in your pathology report will help guide doctors in evaluating the best treatment for you. Remember that some triple-negative cancers are highly aggressive, but others are not. All characteristics of the tumor should be considered. Larger tumors and those with affected lymph nodes require more treatment than smaller, node-negative cancers. The most aggressive treatment is saved for cancer with distant metastases—that is, cancer that has spread to sites beyond the breast and nodes. Researchers have been testing a variety of combinations and are finding more and more options for hormone-negative breast cancer. Some of the most common combinations:

   Adjuvant (after surgery) therapy with ACT: Advances since the 1980s in chemotherapy after surgery—adjuvant therapy—have reduced the risk of death in estrogen-negative patients with affected lymph nodes by 55 percent, according to research published in *JAMA: The Journal of the American Medical Association* (2006).[16] This reduction in death risk translates to a five-year overall survival rate of 83 percent for estrogen-negative, compared to 66 percent for earlier treatment. The benefits of these advances to women with estrogen-positive were negligible.

   Researchers analyzed data from 1985 through 1999 and compared newer regimens of chemotherapy (high-doses of Cytoxan and Adriamycin every two weeks plus Taxol) with older forms (low-doses of Cytoxan and Adriamycin plus fluorouracil every three weeks).

Adjuvant (after surgery) therapy with TAC: Early stage (stage II) triple-negative breast cancer that has progressed to the lymph nodes responded well to a TAC regimen of docetaxel, Adriamycin, and Cytoxan in a 2009 study of 1,350 patients from the Breast Cancer International Research Group (BCIRG) 001 trial. Of these, 14.5 percent were triple-negative. The three-year disease-free survival rate on TAC was 67 percent.[17]

Neoadjuvant (before surgery) therapy with PET: Later stage (node-positive, stage II or III) triple-negative tumors responded well to eight weekly doses before surgery of cisplatin, epirubicin, and Taxol in a phase II trial on patients treated between May 1999 and May 2008 in Naples, Italy, according to a report published in the *Annals of Oncology* (2009). All had large, operable tumors that had spread to the lymph nodes. Seventy-four women received PET plus granulocyte colony-stimulating factor support, which stimulates bone marrow production. Within three weeks of chemo, all had surgery, primarily breast-conserving surgery. Forty-six of the women (62 percent) had a pathologically complete response; the five-year disease-free survival for these women was projected at 90 percent. Disease-free survival for those without a pathologically complete response was 56 percent. This was aggressive treatment, with serious side effects—31 of the patients had severe neutropenia (low white blood count) and anemia (low red blood count).[18]

Neoadjuvant (before surgery) PET plus 5-fluorouracil: Paclitaxel followed by Adriamycin, Cytoxan, plus 5-fluorouracil was effective in preoperative chemo for basal-like tumors. These tumors had a higher rate of pathologically complete response—45 percent—than hormone-positive cancers, which had a 6 percent response. The research, published in *Clinical Cancer Research* (2005), included genetic profiling of 82 breast cancer tumors.[19]

Adjuvant versus neoadjuvant 5-fluorouracil, epirubicin, and cisplatin: The combination of these two anthracyclines plus a platinum agent was effective against triple-negative breast cancer in a study of 541 patients who had been treated between1991 to 2006 at the Royal Marsden Hospital in London. Nineteen percent of the patients—103—were identified as triple-negative. Another 155 had locally recurring or metastatic cancer; of these, 22 percent, or 34 patients, were triple-negative.

Response rates for neoadjuvant chemotherapy were significantly higher for triple-negative tumors (88 percent) than others (51 percent) in research published in *Annals of Oncology* (2008). The five-year overall survival for TNBC tumors following both adjuvant and neoadjuvant chemotherapy, however, was lower—64 percent compared with 85 percent for others. Five-year disease-free survival for TNBC tumors was also lower—57 percent compared with 72 percent for others. Patients with advanced breast cancer had a better overall response rate—41 percent for TNBC tumors and 31 percent for others. Patients with TNBC tumors had a progression-free survival of six months compared with four months for others, although the overall survival was not significantly different between the two groups (11 versus seven months).[20]

Cisplatin: Lab tests comparing cisplatin, doxorubicin, cyclophosphamide, and docetaxel on breast tumors showed that cisplatin was most effective against triple-negative breast cancer.[21] In general, estrogen-negative breast cancer is more sensitive to cisplatin than estrogen-positive and Her2-negative is slightly more sensitive than Her2-positive. Researchers also noted that breast tumors defined as "poorly differentiated" are more sensitive to cisplatin than moderate and well- differentiated tumors. Their conclusion: "Cisplatin is the most active of the four tested drugs in TNBC."

Cisplatin may also be especially effective against triple-negative cancer related to the BRCA1 gene according to research in *Journal of Clinical Oncology* (2010). Researchers treated 28 women with stage II or III TNBC with four cycles of cisplatin every 21 days. The women then had surgery and radiation, based on the assessment of their individual doctors. Of the 28 women, six achieved pathologically complete response. This included women with the BRCA1 gene. Eighteen had a partial response, also a positive sign for long-term health. Four showed a progression of the disease. Younger women showed a better response to the drug, as did women with the BRCA1 mutation.[22]

Paclitaxel plus bevacizumab: This treatment pairs the taxane paclitaxel (Taxol) with the biological agent bevacizumab (Avastin). In phase III clinical trials conducted by the Eastern Cooperative Oncology Group (ECOG) and published in *Journal of Clinical Oncology* (2009), this combination doubled the median progression-free survival over paclitaxel alone. Patients with triple-negative disease benefited more than did those with hormone-positive.[23]

TC: Paclitaxel and carboplatin: In a 2007 retrospective analysis, metastatic triple-negative patients responded well to paclitaxel and carboplatin, even those who had previously been treated with taxanes.[24]

Ixempra plus Xeloda: This combination doubled the progression-free survival (PFS) rate for women with triple-negative breast cancer, according to a study in *Breast Cancer Research and Treatment* (2010) that analyzed the results of five phase II and two phase III studies. In all, 2,261 patients were evaluated, with 24.5 percent, or 556, of these having triple-negative. Women with TNBC who used both Ixempra and Xeloda saw an overall response rate of 23 to 31 percent, with results varying from study to study.

The pathologic complete response for TNBC women on Ixempra was 26 percent, versus 15 percent in the non-triple-negative population.

Patients with metastatic breast cancer in the studies had a variety of treatments before Ixempra therapy, so their overall response rate varied significantly, from 6 to 55 percent; rates, though, were comparable to those in patients with non-triple-negative breast cancer. Progression-free survival was significantly longer for triple-negative patients treated with Ixempra and Xeloda (4.2 months) compared with treatment with Xeloda alone (1.7 months).[25]

EGFR inhibitors: Results on these drugs for breast cancer have been mixed, with one recent phase II clinical trial showing no reduction in breast tumors treated with EGFR.[26] Adding a platinum agent to an EGFR inhibitor, however, showed more success—the EGFR inhibitor cetuximab plus the platinum agent cisplatin doubled the response rate in women with metastatic triple-negative.[27]

On the Horizon

Triple-negative has gained the attention of top researchers around the world. The following are a few of the things they are discovering.

PARP inhibitors: These drugs are being tested for metastatic triple-negative, with some studies showing great hope, especially effective against cancers related to the BRCA mutations; other results, though, have been disappointing. PARP inhibitors block the Poly (ADP-ribose) polymerase pathway, which is important to the development of cancer cells.

Adding the PARP inhibitor Iniparib to chemotherapy added five months to overall survival of patients with metastatic triple-negative breast cancer in a study of 123 women. What's even better is that complete or partial response or stable disease was achieved in 55.7 percent of the women, compared with chemotherapy alone.[28]

But a phase III trial on 519 patients showed no effects on metastatic triple-negative—Iniparib did not increase overall survival or progression-free survival in these patients, despite positive results from the phase II trial.[29]

The debate continues, which will be ultimately resolved with continued clinical trials.

Eribulin: This microtubule inhibitor, still in the experimental stage, improved outcomes of all metastatic breast cancer patients, but was most effective against hormone-negative in a phase III clinical trial in Europe reported in *Journal of Clinical Oncology* (2010). Estrogen- and progesterone-receptor negative patients receiving Eribulin rather than the physician's standard choice of chemotherapy had a 34 percent decreased relative risk of death.[30]

Arsenic: Arsenic trioxide combined with nanotechnology might provide the double whammy that can fight triple-negative breast cancers, according to researchers at Northwestern University. Arsenic has been effective against blood cancers but not against solid tumors because it flushes through the bloodstream too quickly. An arsenic nanoparticle, however, was successful in targeting TNBC in mice, causing cancer cells to die.[31]

Reprogramming TNBC cells to respond to tamoxifen: Researchers at the Samuel Waxman Cancer Research Foundation are studying ways to make triple-negative cells sensitive to tamoxifen.[32] They created a genetic decoy that interfered with protein binding in triple-negative cancer cells, reducing their growth by 80 percent. They see this as the potential for a drug targeted to triple-negative breast cancer.

TNBC vaccine: In 2012, Vaxon Biotech plans to start stage III trials of Vx-001, a vaccine that may be effective against triple-negative breast cancer, with potential availability by 2020.[33]

Insulin-based drugs: Because the insulin-like growth factor receptor IGF-1R may be overexpressed in many cases of triple-negative, several researchers are evaluating this as a route to new drugs for TNBC.

Sorafenib plus cisplatin and paclitaxel: A phase II clinical trial at Emory University is following this combination for triple-negative breast cancer. It includes a preoperative combination of Sorafenib and cisplatin followed by paclitaxel. One goal is to shrink large tumors so they can they be treated with a lumpectomy, rather than a mastectomy.

ACE inhibitors and beta-blockers: According to a study published *in Breast Cancer Research and Treatment* (2011), ACE (angiotensin-converting enzyme) inhibitors may increase the risk of cancer recurrence, but beta-blockers may reduce it. Used together, they can cumulatively reduce risk. Ace inhibitors are used for reducing blood pressure, treating heart failure, preventing strokes, and moderating kidney damage. Beta-blockers treat abnormal heart rhythms, angina, high blood pressure, and migraines.

These results come from lab research on mice, so the effects on humans still need to be studied. If beta-blockers are effective in humans, this could lead to an effective treatment for TNBC. And the study shows that we should evaluate all our medicines, as our drugs affect our entire bodies. The research was based on data from the Life After Cancer Epidemiology (LACE) study of 1,779 patients diagnosed with early-stage breast cancer.[34]

Nuts and Bolts

Websites for Cancer Drug Info
The Internet is full of data on chemo and other cancer drugs. The following sites have solid research behind them.

American Cancer Society Guide to Drugs (http://www.cancer.org). A good overview of drugs for all types of cancer, with side effects, uses, and precautions. The site also has a section on "Complementary and Alternative Methods for Cancer Management."

Breastcancer.org (http://breastcancer.org). In addition to information on chemotherapy drugs, this site has a good discussion on "Types of Complementary Techniques."

Chemocare (http://chemocare.com). With content provided by the Cleveland Clinic Cancer Center, this site was motivated by Scott Hamilton's fight against cancer. It is all about chemo—thorough and easy to navigate. It has a great section on "Complementary Medicine."

Drugs.com (http://www.drugs.com). An independent drug information site with data from Wolters Kluwer Health, American Society of Health-System Pharmacists, Cerner Multum, and Thomson Reuters Micromedex.

Mayo Clinic (http://www.mayoclinic.com). Fueled by research at the Mayo Clinic and elsewhere, with comprehensive, easy-to-digest information.

MedicineNet (http://www.medicinenet.com). Owned and operated by WebMD, with illustrated data on diseases and their cures.

MedlinePlus (http://www.nlm.nih.gov/medlineplus). Provided by the National Institutes of Health and the National Library of Medicine, with information on drugs and supplements for a wide variety of illnesses and disorders.

National Cancer Institute Drug Dictionary (http://cancer.gov/drugdictionary). Quick paragraphs about cancer drugs.

The Rest of You

Oncologists focus on our breast cancer tumors—which is their job—but they often overlook the importance of the rest of the body, says Julie K. Silver, M.D., author of *After Cancer Treatment: Heal Faster, Better, Stronger*. After her bout with breast cancer—she is now more than five years cancer-free—Silver, a physiologist, began focusing on helping cancer patients and survivors thrive through physical activity as part of her oncology rehabilitation emphasis. She offers three keys to health after breast cancer: Exercise regularly, eat a healthy diet, and get enough rest.

I interviewed Julie for a magazine article on breast cancer, and while she talked with me, she took advantage of her telephone time: She hopped onto her elliptical trainer. She says she did this throughout chemotherapy: "I didn't change shoes or clothes. I just exercised in whatever I had on." She didn't feel up to long calls, so sometimes she trained only a few minutes. Eventually, as she got stronger, the calls got longer, until she worked out for a full 30 to 45 minutes.

Some tips that have worked for Julie and her patients—and me:

Walk. Cardiovascular exercise such as regular walks is essential for rebuilding health. If you don't feel strong enough, follow the lead of professional athletes and practice interval training: Cut the walk into smaller parts and rest between each one. I planned my daily walks around the benches in my favorite park; when I got tired, I sat down and watched others walk by. As I recovered, I was able to pass one bench up, and then another, feeling a sense of accomplishment when I made two miles bench-free. I never tried to walk on a chemo day, but the day after I was out hitting the asphalt. Thankfully, I had a husband, children, and siblings to keep me company. We'll explore the benefits of physical activity in chapter 6.

Eat enough. Three small-to-medium meals and two snacks a day will help fight fatigue and maintain balanced blood sugar levels. Emphasize plant-based foods, especially those with dark colors, and limit meat and dairy products. Eat organic whenever possible. (You'll find more about the best foods to eat in the next chapter.)

Rest. Get at least seven hours of sleep a night. If you have trouble sleeping, don't nap during the day. Take rest breaks instead: Read a magazine, go for a scenic drive, or sit on the deck and watch the birds.

BOX 5–5   **Aspirin May Reduce Risk of Recurrence**

Breast cancer patients—regardless of hormone receptor status—who took a low-dose aspirin two to five days a week were 60 percent less likely to have a recurrence and 71 percent less likely to die from breast cancer.

Researchers at Brigham and Women's Hospital in Boston studied data from 4,164 female nurses in the Nurses' Health Study who were diagnosed with breast cancer between 1976 and 2002. By 2006, there had been 400 recurrences and 341 deaths among the nurses.

The findings:

- The majority of women took 81 mg a day, usually for their heart.
- Taking aspirin once a week produced no benefit.
- Tylenol or acetaminophen provided no benefit.
- Both hormone-negative and hormone-positive women benefited.
- Results were essentially the same regardless of stage, menopausal status, or body mass index.

The interpretation:

- Doctors believe aspirin's benefit may come from its anti-inflammatory properties.

The warning:

- The data so far show an association, not a cause, and other factors could be at work, such as the fact that the women who took the aspirin might be more health-conscious than those who did not take aspirin.
- If you have a health problem that can be exacerbated by aspirin, such as ulcers, visit your doctor before considering this approach.
- Aspirin can interfere with the chemotherapy or produce side effects, so check with your doctor if you are undergoing treatment.

Source: Holmes, M. D., Chen, W. Y. Li, L. Hertzmark, E., Spiegelman, D. and Hankinson, S. E. "Aspirin intake and survival after breast cancer," *Journal of Clinical Oncology, vol.* 28, no. 9, 1467–1472 (2011), http://jco.ascopubs.org/content/28/9/1467.full.

Managing Your Emotions

Cancer affects us psychologically, and we need to address it likewise. That means surrounding yourself with friends and family and letting people help you. It is important to be strong, but essential also to acknowledge your needs—you are frightened, perhaps confused, and worried about everything from your disease to your kids, your job, your marriage, your budget.

Friends can truly help keep you grounded.

In fact, researchers at the University of Chicago say social isolation can be a factor in triple-negative breast cancer.[35] They found that women living in a high-crime area of Chicago were more likely to develop triple-negative than other forms of breast cancer. Loneliness and a lack of social outlets, they say, lead to a surge in the stress hormone *cortisol*, which allows tumor cells to grow through efficient use of sugar and fat. But women with a strong social network were more likely to fight against stress, therefore empowering them to combat disease.

Make 'Em Laugh

Dealing with cancer seldom involves a laughfest. Still, a little mirth is good for the soul—and, perhaps, bad for the big "C" cells. Whatever the case, laughing makes us feel better. According to the American Cancer Society, "Although available scientific evidence does not support claims that laughter can cure cancer or any other disease, it can reduce stress and enhance a person's quality of life. Humor has physical effects because it can stimulate the circulatory system, immune system, and other systems in the body."[36]

I come from a family that values humor, so laughing during treatment—and about treatment—was important to me. In fact, when I mentioned to a young friend that I was writing a book on breast cancer, she said, "You should call it *The Funny Book About Breast Cancer*," because she just assumed humor would be part of whatever I did.

And, really, this all is hard enough. Letting yourself laugh is just a blessing.

Cancer centers around the world agree. For example, the MD Anderson Cancer Center, the Kellogg Cancer Center in Chicago, and the Makati Medical Center in the Philippines have all scheduled Laughter Yoga sessions as for patients, health-care staff, and the community.[37] Laughter Yoga—often abbreviated LYoga—combines yogic deep breathing with laughter. Proponents say you need no joke or funny picture to laugh—you can simply force a chuckle, which eventually becomes real and spreads to others around you. Google "Cancer Laughter Yoga" and you'll find numerous videos that will make you laugh right now.

And one book I especially valued during treatment was *Cancer Made Me a Shallower Person: A Memoir in Comics*, by Miriam Engelberg. It gave me the permission to laugh in the face of my disease. Engelberg used cartoons and a sharp wit to take us through her diagnosis, treatment, and, sadly, metastasis. She didn't try to be heroic, settling for being real. My favorite line: "Maybe I caused my cancer by being so depressed. That's so depressing." My son gave me this one, understanding his mother's need to laugh, no matter what. I was deeply saddened when Engelberg died in 2006, but her book remains a beautiful and often hilarious legacy.

Alternative Treatments

Alternative treatments were important to me in my battle with breast cancer—during and after treatment. I used Western medicine to fight the disease, but alternative approaches made this fight easier. Here's what I have done to supplement Western treatments of surgery, chemo, and radiation and to maintain my mental health afterward.

Yoga: This gentle, calming exercise can help keep your body and mind in shape. I do a fairly easy morning routine and, occasionally, a slightly more difficult regimen in the afternoon. I love to do yoga—I look forward to it, and I feel transformed after it. Yoga has helped keep me in shape internally and externally.

In fact, a study presented at the American Society of Clinical Oncology meeting in June 2010 showed that yoga improves the sleep patterns of cancer patients, two-thirds of whom report having trouble sleeping. Participants enrolled in a twice-a-week yoga program that included breathing exercises and restorative yoga postures reported sleeping better and feeling less fatigued.[38]

Meditation: Closely tied to yoga, meditation calms me, helps me think clearly and focus, enables me to sleep better, and in general gives me a flat-out Zen feeling. I am especially sensitive to noise and can be a real crank in crowds, growling at people who pop their gum or chew their ice. Cancer stress did not help. Now, after meditation, if I hear a bothersome noise—a neighbor's stereo, for example—I breathe deeply into the noise and eventually I am calmed.

Many cancer centers offer meditation to patients as a way to reduce stress, improve sleep, even fight pain. The American Cancer Society offers an overview of research on meditation and cancer, noting that meditation can "help to improve the quality of life for people with cancer."[39]

I use a DVD that combines yoga and meditation. One big thing it has taught me is the importance of deep breathing. It is amazing how much better you feel when you let your body fill with oxygen—sort of like a natural antioxidant.

Before cancer I used to love my evening drink—or drinks: a martini, perhaps followed by a couple glasses of wine. I used alcohol to relax me. No more. One meditation session relaxes me way more than alcohol ever did—and the benefits continue, whereas alcohol-induced relaxation turns to nervousness and sleeplessness. So if yoga and meditation do nothing more than reduce my drinking, they have provided a serious benefit.

Acupuncture: Research, mostly in China where acupuncture originated, demonstrates that acupuncture can reduce nausea, vomiting, and pain.[40]

My acupuncturist is a wonder. I went to her before each chemotherapy session, and she prepared me well and, I believe, reduced my stress as well as my nausea. Now, she has a perceptive link to my health that truly balances me. I can walk into Abby's office feeling internally whacky and leave feeling truly connected to my health. I have gone to her for allergies, poison ivy, lingering colds, joint pain, and anything else that has not responded to my normal ministrations. When she listens to my pulse, she hears everything from the fact that I have recently eaten nuts and not chewed them thoroughly enough to the stomach upset I hadn't yet mentioned. I believe that if I had a serious health problem, she would be plugged into it before I was. She wouldn't be able to diagnose it, of course, but she would know something was off and send me to a doctor to be checked.

And, really, if *all* she does is relax me, she is magic.

Guided imagery: This can help reduce depression and may even offer a boost to the immune system.[41] I did it on my own, but I think working with a therapist would make it better. At night, I would envision my cancer; then I would envision a white light eating it away. Once, I got an image of a PacMan chomping the cancer out. That made me smile, which was a nice side effect.

Prayer: A friend once quipped, "There are no atheists in the chemo ward." I suspect there are, and that prayer has to be defined fairly broadly. But asking for help beyond yourself can be life-affirming and can make you see beyond your own ills. I did use plain old prayer. I visited the cathedral downtown, a quiet, meditative space. I always lit a candle to my parents and asked for their help—I lost both of them to cancer. And then I went into a pew and prayed a short prayer, then recited my mantra, with deep breaths—*health in, sickness out, health in, sickness out.* My health did come in, my sickness did go out.

Follow-Up Care After Hormone-Negative Breast Cancer

"I feel fine. I hope I am fine. I like to live like I'm fine," Deb Lowman-Melchionda told me as she approached the second anniversary of her diagnosis. She was 42 when she was diagnosed with triple-negative in December 2008—a 1.2-centimeter tumor with no affected lymph nodes.

She had no family history of breast cancer—"I have no idea where this came from," she says. She used birth control pills and had fertility treatments for in vitro fertilization, so she wonders about those effects. She is part Puerto Rican, so her Hispanic heritage could also have had an influence.

This mother of two—her sons were 4 and 9 when she was diagnosed—calls herself a natural worrier. She dreads her regular blood tests for cancer markers because, she says, "I want a break. If anything came up on a test, I would just lose it."

She found the lump herself—she'd had one mammogram when she turned 40, but kept putting off the second.

I had noticed over the past few months that when I laid down flat on my stomach I had a pain in the underside of my right breast. Since I'd always had sore breasts off and on due to menstrual cycles, pregnancy, breast-feeding, it didn't seem significant and I chalked it up to hormones. But then one day in the shower I decided to do a self-exam because of the pain and was shocked to find a lump. It was one of those world-just-dropped moments—I immediately panicked and thought the worst. And in this case, I was right.

I had done self-exams at other points in the past, mostly whenever I thought of it. But I also have dense breasts with lots of little palpable bumps, so it seemed rather useless at times. However, there was no mistaking this lump—it turned out to be 1.2 centimeters.

Deb, a 3-D computer animator from Atlanta, Georgia, had a lumpectomy and an axillary node dissection, followed by 12 weeks of chemo with Adriamycin, Cytoxan, and Taxol.

Then came another blow—tests revealed DCIS in the same breast, so she had a double mastectomy followed by reconstruction. She now takes a bone-strengthening drug every six months.

Since treatment, she has been trying to exercise a half-hour five days a week. She's focusing on her diet—five servings of fruits and vegetables a day, with blueberries every morning, an orange a day, plus baby aspirin and vitamin D3, omega 3s, and vitamins E supplements.

But still she worries.

"I don't want my kids to grow up without a mommy," she says. "I'm terrified of tests now."

Her doctor persuaded her to see a psychiatrist as her worry and anxiety were taking over her life. She's now on an antidepressant, which, she says, has helped. "I no longer obsess as much as I used to about every little symptom, though the fear is still there. I have been able to enjoy my life once again."

Much of Deb's stress was related to the bevy of tests we undergo for cancer follow-up—mammograms, chest X-rays, blood markers. In many cases, follow-up care is more stressful than the actual breast cancer treatment itself. At least during treatment, we had something of a sense of progress and the hope that we would be cured and that this disease would be behind us. Plus our focus was on getting through one thing at a time.

After we slow down and have time to think, we ask, "What the heck happened here?"

Follow-up care, however, reminds us that the disease still could lurk, that what happened once could happen again. And the second time it could be worse. So our anxiety level often spikes when we are due for our regular follow-up exams.

And, it appears, many of us are tested too much.

The American Society of Clinical Oncology (ASCO) guidelines recommend a simple approach—a regular physical exam plus breast imaging. The exam, they say, should include a careful history and should be done by a "physician experienced in the surveillance of cancer patients and in breast examination."[42] That does not mean it has to be an oncologist—it could be a primary care physician or even a physician's assistant.

ASCO recommends meeting with a physician every three to six months for the first three years and every six to 12 months in years four and five. And this is just for the physical exam and an evaluation of your history and symptoms. They specifically note that they do **not** recommend blood testing, bone scans, chest X-rays, liver ultrasounds, or computer tomography in patients with no symptoms.

Women who have had breast conservation surgery—a lumpectomy—should have regular breast imaging once a year; this is usually mammography, but it can be an MRI in special cases.

Because triple-negative breast cancer can grow quickly, doctors often order mammograms twice a year for the first three years.

Those who have had reconstructive surgery should not need additional mammograms—a comprehensive regular physical exam should provide adequate surveillance.[43]

Profile

Cancer Brings Love the Second Time Around

Rosa Martin DuPree knows all about hope—that and faith are her job. She is a Baptist minister in Hampton, Virginia, where she started an outreach ministry in 1992, counseling those who have lost a loved one, serving food to shut-ins, and visiting a nursing home with Alzheimer's patients. "They call me Ms. Sunshine," she says.

And she needed that attitude when she met what she calls the Red Devil—a nickname some give to Adriamycin because of its red color and its aftereffects. Others call it the Red Death. Rosa's doctors used Adriamycin, Cytoxan, and Taxol to fight triple-negative breast cancer, essentially the same drugs as Sheri was on, although Rosa had chemo after surgery, whereas Sheri had chemo before surgery. Rosa was diagnosed in March 2008 at 59 with a 3.3-centimeter tumor but no affected lymph nodes. Her chemo was preceded by a lumpectomy and followed by radiation.

Risk factors? She is African-American and was on Premarin for 9 years, although hormone-replacement therapy (HRT) is more related to hormone-positive breast cancer.

She has had no signs of recurrence, but the side effects were significant: "Of course I lost all of my hair. I didn't gain my full strength and energy level for over 18 months. My white blood counts stayed low for months. And still, every night at 9 p.m.—I don't care where I am—my body shuts down. I can no longer function. My entire body stiffens. I get the help of my husband to get me to bed and, once in bed, I need his assistance to turn from side to side. I use a cane sometimes for support, taking away the possibility of a fall. I cannot over exert myself, or I have to rest the next day."

She has not told her physician about her weakness, largely because she doesn't want the drugs she knows he will recommend.

"I don't share everything with the doctor unless it's something I can't handle," she says. "The doctors are quick to write a prescription to medicate whatever. I don't really want a lot of meds with long-term effects put into my body. So I find comfort in over-the-counter Aleve, I drink teas to relax me, I massage myself, and I let hubby massage me. I find my positive attitude toward life keeps me feeling good and gives me the determination to live, laugh, love, and encourage others along their way."

She's big on reading all she can about triple-negative breast cancer, so she heads to the doctor well prepared. "When he talks with me I've already researched the pill, the complaint, and what it can do for me."

When I first interviewed Rosa, she was just Rosa Martin. But on September 16, 2010, two and a half years after diagnosis, she married "a jewel of a sweetheart," William DuPree. He had actually proposed before she was diagnosed, but she was hesitant. She had spent 20 years caring for a psychologically abusive bipolar husband who had died four years earlier. She wasn't ready to jump back into the frying pan, and she was afraid to entirely trust that William was a totally different type of man.

What happened to change her mind? Cancer, and the fact that William took loving care of her throughout treatment. Her two children, in their late 30s, lived out of state, so it was up to William to give Rosa the care she needed. And, boy, did he. "He fed me, he sat with me when I had my treatments, and when he couldn't, he made sure I got there safely. He shopped for food, put money in my account, bought me things of my heart. I love perfume and he made sure I got what I wanted."

He loved her not only in words, she says. "He loved me in deed."

Notes

1. Fisher, Bernard, Anderson, Stewart, Bryant, John, Margolese, Richard G., Deutsch, Melvin, Fisher, Jeong, Jong-Hyeon, and Wolmark, Norman, "Twenty-year follow-up of a randomized trial comparing total mastectomy, lumpectomy, and lumpectomy plus irradiation for the treatment of invasive breast cancer," *New England Journal of Medicine*, vol. 347, 1233–1241 (2002). Find the full article at http://www.cinj.org/documents/TotalmastectomyvsLumpectomy.pdf.
2. For Deborah's self-portrait, go to *Love, Cancer, Etc.*, at http://ddlatt.blogspot.com/search/label/after%20cancer.
3. Bedrosian, Isabelle, Hu, Chung-Yuan, and Chang, George J., "Population-based study of contralateral prophylactic mastectomy and survival outcomes of breast cancer patients," *Journal of the National Cancer Institute*, vol. 102, no. 6, 401–409 (2010).
4. Neuman, Heather B., Morrogh, Mary, Gonen, Mithat, Van Zee, Kimberly J., Morrow, Monica, and King, Tari A., "Stage IV breast cancer in the era of targeted therapy," *Cancer*, vol. 116, no. 5, 1226–1233 (2010).

5. Rebbeck, Timothy R., Kauff, Noah D., and Domchek, Susan M., "Meta-analysis of risk reduction estimates associated with risk-reducing salpingo-oophorectomy in BRCA1 or BRCA2 mutation carriers," *Journal of the National Cancer Institute*, vol. 101, no. 2, 80–87 (2009).

6. Giuliano, Armando E., Hunt, Kelly K., Ballman, Karla V., Beitsch, Peter D., Whitworth, Pat W., Blumencranz, Peter W., Leitch, A. Marilyn, Saha, Sukamal, McCall, Linda M., and Morrow, Monica, "Axillary dissection vs no axillary dissection in women with invasive breast cancer and sentinel node metastasis," *JAMA: The Journal of the American Medical Association*, vol. 305, no. 6, 569–575 (2011).

7. Petit, T., Wilt, M., Velten, M., Millon, R., Rodier, J-F F., Borel, C., Mors, R., Haegelé, P., Eber, M., and Ghnassia, J-P P., "Comparative value of tumour grade, hormonal receptors, Ki-67, HER-2 and topoisomerase II alpha status as predictive markers in breast cancer patients treated with neoadjuvant anthracycline-based chemotherapy," *European Journal of Cancer*, vol. 40, no. 2, 205–211 (2004).

8. Bonilla, Luisa, Ben-Aharon, Irit, Vidal, Liat, Gafter-Gvili, Anat, Leibovici, Leonard, and Stemmer, Salomon M., "Dose-dense chemotherapy in nonmetastatic breast cancer: a systematic review and meta-analysis of randomized controlled trials," *Journal of the National Cancer Institute*, vol. 102, no. 24, 1845–1854 (2010). For the full article, go to http://jnci.oxfordjournals.org/content/early/2010/11/23/jnci.djq409.full.

9. De Giorgi, U., Rosti, G., Frassineti, L., Kopf, B., Giovannini, N., Zumaglini, F., and Marangolo, M., "High-dose chemotherapy for triple negative breast cancer," *Annals of Oncology*, vol. 18, no. 1, 202–203 (2007). For the full article, go to http://annonc.oxfordjournals.org/content/18/1/202.full.

10. Sparano, Joseph A., Wang, Molin, Martino, Silvana, Jones, Vicky, Perez, Edith A., Saphner, Tom, Wolff, Antonio C., Sledge, George W., Wood, William C., and Davidson, Nancy E., "Weekly paclitaxel in the adjuvant treatment of breast cancer," *New England Journal of Medicine*, vol. 358, no. 16, 1663–1671 (2008). For the full article, go to http://www.nejm.org/doi/pdf/10.1056/NEJMoa0707056.

11. von Minckwitz, Gunter, Eidtmann, Holger, Rezai, Mahdi, Fasching, Peter A., Tesch, Hans, Eggemann, Holm, Schrader, Iris, Kittel, Kornelia, Hanusch, Claus, Kreienberg, Rolf, Solbach, Christine, Gerber, Bernd, Jackisch, Christian, Kunz, Georg, Blohmer, Jens-Uwe, Huober, Jens, Hauschild, Maik, Fehm, Tanja, Müller, Berit M., Denkert, Carsten, Loibl, Sibylle, Nekljudova, Valentina, and Untch, Michael, "Neoadjuvant chemotherapy and bevacizumab for HER2-negative breast cancer," *New England Journal of Medicine*, vol. 366, no. 4, 299–309 (2012).

12. Bear, Harry D., Tang, Gong, Rastogi, Priya, Geyer, Charles E., Robidoux, André, Atkins, James N., Baez-Diaz, Luis, Brufsky, Adam M., Mehta, Rita S., Fehrenbacher, Louis, Young, James A., Senecal, Francis M., Gaur, Rakesh, Margolese, Richard G., Adams, Paul T., Gross, Howard M., Costantino, Joseph P., Swain, Sandra M., Mamounas, Eleftherios P., and Wolmark, Norman, "Bevacizumab added to neoadjuvant chemotherapy for breast cancer," *New England Journal of Medicine*, vol. 366, no. 4, 310–320 (2012).

13. Pritchard, Kathleen I., "Tailored targeted therapy for all: a realistic and worthwhile objective against," *Breast Cancer Research*, vol. 11, Suppl. 3 (2009).

14. Li, C. I., Daling, J. R., Porter, P. L., Tang, M. C., and Malone, K. E., "Adjuvant hormonal therapy for breast cancer and risk of hormone receptor-specific subtypes of contralateral breast cancer," *Cancer Research*, vol. 69, no. 17, 6865–6870 (2009). For the full article, go to http://www.ncbi.nlm.nih.gov/pmc/articles/PMC2745902/.

15. Sabnis, G., and Brodie, A., "Trastuzumab sensitizes ER negative, HER-2 positive breast cancer cells (SKBr-3) to endocrine therapy," *ENDO* 2009; Abstract OR38–02.

16. Berry, Donald A., Cirrincione, Constance, Henderson, I. Craig, Citron, Marc L., Budman, Daniel R., Goldstein, Lori J., Martino, Silvana, Perez, Edith A., Muss, Hyman B., Norton, Larry, Hudis, Clifford, and Winer, Eric P., "Estrogen-receptor status and outcomes of modern chemotherapy for patients with node-positive breast cancer," *JAMA: The Journal of the American Medical Association*, vol. 295, no. 14, 1658–1667 (2006). For the full article, go to http://www.ncbi.nlm.nih.gov/pmc/articles/PMC1459540/.

17. Hugh, Judith, Hanson, John, Cheang, Maggie C., Nielsen, Torsten O., Perou, Charles M., Dumontet, Charles, Reed, John, Krajewska, Maryla, Treilleux, Isabelle, Rupin, Matthieu, Magherini, Emmanuelle, Mackey, John, Martin, Miguel, and Vogel, Charles, "Breast cancer subtypes and response to docetaxel in node-positive breast cancer: use of an immunohistochemical definition in the BCIRG 001 trial," *Journal of Clinical Oncology*, vol. 27, no. 8, 1168–1176 (2009).

18. Frasci, G., Comella, P., Rinaldo, M., Iodice, G., Di Bonito, M., D'Aiuto, M., Petrillo, A., Lastoria, S., Siani, C., Comella, G., and D'Aiuto, G., "Preoperative weekly cisplatin–epirubicin–paclitaxel with G-CSF support in triple-negative large pperable breast cancer," *Annals of Oncology*, vol. 20, no. 7, 1185–1192 (2009). For the full article, go to http://annonc.oxfordjournals.org/content/20/7/1185.full.

19. Rouzier, Roman, Perou, Charles M., Symmans, W. Fraser, Ibrahim, Nuhad, Cristofanilli, Massimo, Anderson, Keith, Hess, Kenneth R., Stec, James, Ayers, Mark, Wagner, Peter, Morandi, Paolo, Fan, Chang, Rabiul, Islam, Ross, Jeffrey S., Hortobagyi, Gabriel N., and Pusztai, Lajos, "Breast cancer molecular subtypes respond differently to preoperative chemotherapy," *Clinical Cancer Research*, vol. 11, no. 16, 5678–5685 (2005).

20 Sirohi, B., Arnedos, M., Popat, S., Ashley, S., Nerurkar, A., Walsh, G., Johnston, S., and Smith, I. E., "Platinum-based chemotherapy in triple-negative breast cancer," *Annals of Oncology*, vol. 19, no. 11, 1847–1852 (2008).

21. Weisenthal, L., "Activity of cisplatin in triple-negative breast cancer in comparison to other cancer types in fresh tumor cell culture assay using a cell death endpoint," Annual Meeting, American Society of Clinical Oncology, San Francisco (2009).

22. Silver, Daniel P., Richardson, Andrea L., Eklund, Aron C., Wang, Zhigang C., Szallasi, Zoltan, Li, Qiyuan, Juul, Nicolai, Leong, Chee-Onn, Calogrias, Diana, Buraimoh, Ayodele, Fatima, Aquila, Gelman, Rebecca S., Ryan, Paula D., Tung, Nadine M., De Nicolo, Arcangela, Ganesan, Shridar, Miron, Alexander, Colin, Christian, Sgroi, Dennis C., Ellisen, Leif W., Winer, Eric P., and Garber, Judy E., "Efficacy of neoadjuvant cisplatin in triple-negative breast cancer," *Journal of Clinical Oncology*, vol. 28, no. 7, 1145–1153 (2010).

23. Gray, Robert, Bhattacharya, Suman, Bowden, Christopher, Miller, Kathy, and Comis, Robert L., "Independent review of E2100: a phase III trial of bevacizumab plus paclitaxel versus paclitaxel in women with metastatic breast cancer," *Journal of Clinical Oncology*, vol. 27, no. 30, 4966–4972 (2009).

24. Chia, J. W., Ang, P., See, H., Wong, Z., Soh, L., Yap, Y., and Wong, N., "Triple-negative metastatic/recurrent breast cancer: treatment with paclitaxel/carboplatin combination chemotherapy," *Journal of Clinical Oncology (Meeting Abstracts)*, vol. 25, no. 18, Suppl., 1086+ (2007).

25. Perez, Edith, Patel, Tejal, and Moreno-Aspitia, Alvaro, "Efficacy of ixabepilone in ER/PR/HER2-negative (triple-negative) breast cancer," *Breast Cancer Research and Treatment*, vol. 121, no. 2, 261–271 (2010).

26. Green, M. D., Francis, P. A., Gebski, V., Harvey, V., Karapetis, C., Chan, A., Snyder, R., Fong, A., Basser, R., and Forbes, J. F., on behalf of the Australian New Zealand Breast Cancer Trials Group, "Gefitinib treatment in hormone-resistant and hormone receptor-negative advanced breast cancer," *Annals of Oncology*, vol. 20, no. 11, 1813–1817 (2009).

27. Baselga, J., Gomez, P., Awada, A., et al., "The addition of cetuximab to cisplatin increases overall response rate and progression-free survival in metastatic triple-negative breast cancer: results of a randomized phase II study," 35th European Society of Medical Oncologists Congress, Milan, Italy (2010).

28. Nelson, Roxanne, "Iniparib improves survival in metastatic triple-negative breast cancer," *WebMD*, October 10, 2010, http://www.medscape.com/viewarticle/730211 (accessed December 10, 2010).

29. Haley, Shirley, "Disappointing results in study of iniparib for metastatic triple-negative breast cancer," *Internal Medicine News*, January 31, 2011.

30. Twelves, C., Loesch, D., Blum, J. L., Vahdat, L. T., Petrakova, K., Chollet, P. J., Akerele, C. E., Seegobin, S., Wanders, J., and Cortes, J., "A phase III study (EMBRACE) of eribulin mesylate versus treatment of physician's choice in patients with locally recurrent or metastatic breast cancer previously treated with an anthracycline and a taxane," *Journal of Clinical Oncology*, vol. 28, no. 18 suppl., CRA 1004 (2010).

31. Paul, Maria, "New arsenic nanoparticle blocks aggressive breast cancer," press release from Northwestern University, July 15, 2010, http://www.northwestern.edu/newscenter/stories/2010/07/nano particle-blocks-aggressive-breast-cancer.html (accessed December 10, 2010).

32. Farias, Eduardo F., Petrie, Kevin, Leibovitch, Boris, Murtagh, Janice, Chornet, Manuel B., Schenk, Tino, Zelent, Arthur, and Waxman, Samuel, "Interference with Sin3 function induces epigenetic reprogramming and differentiation in breast cancer cells," *Proceedings of the National Academy of Sciences of the United States of America*, vol. 107, no. 26, 11811–11816 (2009).

33. "Vaxon Biotech concludes vaccine trial," *Drug Discovery and Development*, May 27, 2010, http://www.dddmag.com/news-Vaxon-Biotech-Concludes-Vaccine-Trial-51710.aspx (accessed December 12, 2010).

34. Ganz, Patricia A., Habel, Laurel A., Weltzien, Erin K., Caan, Bette J., and Cole, Steven W., "Examining the influence of beta blockers and ACE inhibitors on the risk for breast cancer recurrence: results from the LACE cohort," *Breast Cancer Research and Treatment*, vol. 129, no. 2, 549–556 (2011).

35. Hermes, Gretchen L., Delgado, Bertha, Tretiakova, Maria, Cavigelli, Sonia A., Krausz, Thomas, Conzen, Suzanne D., and McClintock, Martha K., "Social isolation dysregulates endocrine and behavioral stress while increasing malignant burden of spontaneous mammary tumors," *Proceedings of the National Academy of Sciences of the United States of America*, vol. 106, no. 52, 22393–22398 (2009).

36. "Humor therapy," American Cancer Society, http://www.cancer.org/Treatment/TreatmentsandSideEffects/Complementary andAlternativeMedicine/MindBodyandSpirit/humor-therapy (accessed November 10, 2010).

37. Estavillo, Elvie, "Healing laughter with breast cancer survivors," *Philippine Star*, October 26, 2010, http://www.philstar.com/Article.aspx?articleId=624158&publicationSubCategoryId=80 (accessed November 10, 2010).

38. Mustian, K. M., Palesh, O., Sprod, L., Peppone, L. J., Heckler, C. E., Yates, J. S., Reddy, P. S., Melnik, M., Giguere, J. K., and Morrow, G. R., "Effect of YOCAS yoga on sleep, fatigue, and quality of life: a URCC CCOP randomized, controlled clinical trial among

410 cancer survivors," *Journal of Clinical Oncology*, vol. 28, no. 15s (2010).

39. "Meditation," American Cancer Society, http://www.cancer.org/Treatment/TreatmentsandSideEffects/Complementaryand AlternativeMedicine/MindBodyandSpirit/meditation.

40. "Acupuncture," National Cancer Institute, http://www.cancer.gov/cancertopics/pdq/cam/acupuncture/patient/page1.

41. "Guided Imagery," Breastcancer.org, http://www.breastcancer.org/treatment/comp_med/types/imagery.jsp.

42. Find the ASCO Guidelines online at http://www.asco.org.[43.] "Consider variables before imaging reconstructed breast for cancer," *HemOnctoday* (April 25, 2011), http://www.healio.com/Hematology-Oncology/Breast-Cancer/news/print/hematology-oncology/%7BE610AD0E-7C37–4323–8F6F-D9E4597891FE%7D/Consider-variables-before-imaging-reconstructed-breast-for-cancer.

6

The Positives of Healthy Living

HERE'S ONE WAY TO GET OVER THE WORRIES ABOUT cancer treatment and the fears of its return: Run a triathlon or two. That's the approach Julie Desloge took—she completed her first sprint triathlon in June 2010, a little more than two years after she was diagnosed with triple-negative breast cancer. She participated in two additional races that summer—and her radiation oncologist was her teammate on the final one.

On that race, her doctor swam 1.5 kilometers, another friend ran 10 kilometers, and Julie biked 40 kilometers. That translates to slightly less than a mile swim, a 24.8-mile bike ride, and a 6.2-mile run.

Phew!

And a year later, in June 2011, just one week shy of her third cancerversary, Julie finished another race, this time the entire sprint triathlon:

Swimming
Biking
Running
The entire thing.

Double phew!

Julie is thoroughly enjoying her healthy new pursuit and enjoying life, period. It took some doing and a serious commitment—eight months of training that was far from easy. Running, she writes on her blog, is the most difficult for her—she has trouble getting enough air. But she keeps at it and each time it is a little easier.[1]

Julie was diagnosed with a 2.6-centimeter triple-negative tumor in February 2008 when she was 41. She had neoadjuvant chemotherapy—four rounds of Taxotere and Cytoxan—that got rid of all but 0.3 centimeters of the tumor, a nearly 90 percent reduction.

Easily speaking the jargon on cancer, she says, "No pathologically complete response for me." And, while her response was only partial, it nevertheless was significant, offering her a positive prognosis that she is making the most of.

A lumpectomy followed chemo, with radiation after that.

Risk factors? She's negative for the BRCA mutation, but wonders about her reproductive history—she started her periods young, at age 11. And she's the mother of three children, who were 11, nine, and six at the time of diagnosis, although she breast-fed all three for nine to 10 months.

She was about 15 pounds overweight when she was diagnosed. Her weight continues to be a challenge, even with her high level of exercise. She now weighs more than she did at diagnosis, although much of that is probably muscle, which weighs more than fat. "I haven't really found the key to unlocking much weight loss," she says. Still, we're talking about being only slightly beyond her ideal—Julie says her BMI is a healthy 24.8.

She had been exercising regularly before cancer, doing cardio and resistance workouts four to five days a week. But she upped the ante after treatment and hit the sprint triathlon circuit with her husband Denis near their Portland, Oregon, home.

Cancer, she says, not only gave her motivation to maintain a healthy lifestyle, but it provided a chance to look outside herself at what others are going through. She's bothered when friends protest that they should not complain about any problems they encounter, given what she faced in cancer treatment. "Pain is pain," she says.

The one effect she could do without is the constant anxiety that comes from follow-up doctor visits. "While my doctors are incredible people and I enjoy them personally, I still don't like the reason I have to see them," she says.

By making her radiation oncologist her racing partner, she's turning at least one medical relationship into a fun one, helping her move on with her life at a pretty good clip.

Exercise and Physical Activity

I grew up in Colorado and spent much of my life hiking the mountains. I still love to hike, and I do it regularly. I hit a time in my life, however, when responsibilities kept me from regular physical activity. I spent the majority of my workday at a desk or in front of a classroom, where I ambled roughly 10 feet or so from the lectern. Nevertheless, I had full days with little time for breaks, so after work I often ended up exhausted and sleeping on the couch in front of the TV.

My weight crept up and up—an average of five pounds a year—until I was 50 pounds overweight at age 59. I was just shy of obese, with a body mass index of 29.

Fortunately, the yearly physical required by my insurance company set me straight. My numbers—cholesterol, weight, BMI, percentage of body fat, blood sugar—were all dangerously high. And the 20-page report I got after the exam included page after page of the same reminder: *This would be improved if you lost weight.*

Like many overweight people, I had tried to lose the pounds before and always failed. Finally, I took the plunge and hired a personal trainer who motivated me to lose. I was paying him good money, and I had announced to all my friends that I was going to drop the fat. I am far from rich, plus I am generally a cheapskate, so giving somebody money for what might seem like vanity was a real stretch for me. A friend put it into perspective though: "How much do you think a heart attack would cost you?" Neither of us thought of cancer. So I signed up. It took me two years to lose the extra 50 pounds I had gained, and I have kept the weight off ever since. My motivation changed, though. My cancer diagnosis came nine months after I embarked on this healthy regimen.

Would I have dodged the cancer bullet had I kept up the exercise of my adolescence? Maybe. That youthful exercise 40 years before the cancer, though, might have been the reason that I had an easier recovery. And my continuing exercise will, I hope, help keep my cancer from recurring.

I now make sure I have at least four hours weekly of significant physical activity—usually hiking or walking. I consider it part of my continuing cancer therapy. The following studies illustrate why I am now such a fan of exercise.

Body Size, Activity, and TNBC

Postmenopausal women who exercised the most had the lowest incidence of both triple-negative and hormone-positive breast cancer, according to research published in *Cancer Epidemiology, Biomarkers & Prevention* (2011) using data from the Women's Health Initiative on 155,723 women.[2] The same is true of those with the lowest body mass index (BMI): Those least at risk had a BMI of less than 23.75, and those most at risk had a BMI over 31. The effects, researchers said, were modest, but they do point to ways women can control their cancer risks.

BOX 6–1   **Determining Your Body Mass Index**

The body mass index (BMI) is one way of determining how much fat you have in your body. A normal BMI is 18.5 to 24.9. Below that, you are underweight. Between 25 and 29.9, you are overweight; above 30, you are obese. The easiest way to determine your BMI is with an online calculator. If you love math, though, you can calculate your BMI by dividing your weight in pounds by height in inches squared, and multiplying by 703. The Centers for Disease Control and Prevention has an online calculator (http://www.cdc.gov/healthyweight/assessing/bmi/) that is simple to use.

Some problems with the BMI, though: It does not take into account things like body makeup. An athlete who is all muscle could show up as overweight because muscle weighs more than fat. And the dividing points are arbitrary. A 5'6" woman who weighs 154 is in the normal range. When she

Box 6–1 (Continued)

adds a pound, though, she is overweight. Still, the BMI is a good overall gauge.

Height	Weight	BMI	Category
4 feet 10 inches	100–119	21–24.9	Normal
	120–144	25–29.9	Overweight
	Over 145	Over 30	Obese
5 feet 2 inches	110–134	21–24.9	Normal
	135–164	25–29.9	Overweight
	Over 164	Over 30	Obese
5 feet 6 inches	124–154	21–24.9	Normal
	155–184	25–29.9	Overweight
	Over 185	Over 30	Obese
5 feet 10 inches	140–174	21–24.9	Normal
	175–209	25–29.9	Overweight
	Over 210	Over 30	Obese

Long-Term Exercise

The California Teachers Study found that long-term exercise—both strenuous (like running) and moderate (brisk walking)—was associated with reduced risk of estrogen-negative breast cancer. The strongest influence comes from vigorous activity like jogging and with exercise for more than four hours a week, continued for more than a year.[34] Exercise did not affect the risk of estrogen receptor-positive breast cancer. Earlier research found similar results, with the risk of estrogen-negative breast cancer significantly decreasing with physical activity.[5]

Exercise and Younger Women

Research using data from the Nurses Health Study showed that younger women can reduce their cancer risk with exercise. The study, of 64,777 premenopausal women, showed significant benefit from exercise during the teen and young adult years—between 12 and 22.

BOX 6–2   Menopausal Status and Exercise

A study in *Cancer Epidemiology, Biomarkers & Prevention* (2006) found a strong correlation between exercise and reduction in both hormone-positive and hormone-negative disease. Participants aged 25 to 64 were given a questionnaire in which they reported their exercise patterns from adolescence through the 10 years before the interview. The researchers determined the following:

- Exercise in adolescence and within the 10 years before diagnosis was associated with decreased risk of hormone-negative and hormone-positive breast cancers in both premenopausal and postmenopausal women: in short, all cancer, all women.
- Women who exercised reduced their risk by 30 to 60 percent over those who did not exercise. Again, this was true of premenopausal and postmenopausal women.
- Activity during both adolescence and the 10 years before diagnosis resulted in a risk reduction of 62 to 79 percent for hormone-negative breast cancer.
- Postmenopausal women benefited the most from exercise.
- Sweating during exercise in the 10 years before the study was associated with decreased risk for all forms of breast cancer among postmenopausal women. Researchers aren't sure why, but it may be that sweating implies more strenuous exercise.

Source: Adams, S. A., Matthews, C. E., Hebert, J. R., Moore, C. G., Cunningham, J. E., Shu, J. E., Fulton, J., Gao, Y., and Zheng, W., "Association of physical activity with hormone receptor status: the Shanghai Breast Cancer Study," *Cancer Epidemiology, Biomarkers & Prevention*, vol. 15, no. 6, 1170–1178 (2006).

Women 23 to 34 showed a slightly reduced benefit. Women over 35 gained no risk reduction. The best exercise: running 3.25 hours a week or walking 13 hours a week, which brought a 23 percent risk reduction. While researchers did not categorize results based on hormone status, triple-negative breast cancer is most common among premenopausal women. The study was published in the *Journal of the National Cancer Institute* (2008).[6]

Cancer Survivors and Exercise

Breast cancer survivors are among the least physically active cancer survivors, which turns out to be a pretty sedentary group. In a study published in *Cancer* (2008), the journal of the American Cancer Society, Canadian researchers discovered that cancer survivors, for the most part, had a surprisingly unhealthy lifestyle. Among the least active were survivors of colorectal and breast cancer, and female melanoma survivors. The most active: male skin cancer survivors.[7]

Twenty-one percent of the 114,000 Canadians who were interviewed for the study were physically active; 18 percent were obese. By comparison, 25 percent of Canadians are physically active and 15 percent are obese. Breast cancer survivors were only about half as likely to be physically active as women who had not had cancer.

Nuts and Bolts

Exercise: Way to Go
Exercise can eventually become a given in your daily schedule—if you are physically up to it. Weight-loss experts prefer to talk about physical activity rather than exercise, because it is more inclusive and less overwhelming. It includes everything from mowing the lawn to jogging. No matter what you call it, the more you do, and the more strenuous it is, the better.

Start slowly. Overdoing it at the beginning is the biggest mistake people make when starting an exercise regimen. Build up gradually, allowing your body to get accustomed to a new way of life.

Do what you enjoy. Don't decide that you will jog every morning if you truly hate to run. Walk instead. And look for scenery that can help divert your attention. If you are not up to rigorous walks, do what you can.

Exercise early or often. If at all possible, go for that walk first thing in the morning, before the excuses of the day build up and before you're too tired to care. If that doesn't work, add physical activity to your day whenever you can. Maybe a walk after breakfast or playing with the kids or grandkids in the afternoon.

Find a support system. Look for an exercise buddy. Time goes by much quicker if you are jabbering with a friend. Plus, you're more likely to show up for that evening walk if somebody is waiting for you.

Avoid saboteurs. Everybody has an opinion on how you are supposed to do things during and after treatment. Avoid people who aren't positive about your goals.

Weight Control

Perhaps the biggest thing you can do to help your overall health and reduce your risk of cancers of all kinds is to maintain a healthy weight, usually a body mass index (BMI) of under 25, which is 150 pounds for a 5-foot, 5-inch woman.[8,9]

According to the Collaborative Women's Longevity Study, women who gained more than 22 pounds after diagnosis were 83 percent more likely to die of breast cancer than those who stayed within five pounds of their original weight.[10] In fact, women increased their death risk by 14 percent for every 11 pounds they gained after diagnosis. The study, published in *Cancer Epidemiology, Biomarkers & Prevention* (2009), looked at the BMIs of 4,020 breast cancer patients from 1988 to 2001. Those categorized as obese—having a BMI of 30 or above—were 2.5 times more likely to die of breast cancer.

The ongoing Nurses Health Study showed similar results. Women who gained 55 pounds or more after age 18 had almost 1.5 times the risk of breast cancer compared with those who maintained their weight.[11] Researchers studied 121,700 women, all married nurses between 30 to 55 years old, from 1976 to 2002; 4,393 of these ultimately were diagnosed with invasive breast cancer. At special risk were women who gained weight after menopause: Those who gained 22 pounds or more since menopause increased their risk by 1.2 times compared to those who had not gained weight. But a bonus for late-losers like me: Women who lost 22 pounds or more since menopause and kept the weight off were at a lower risk than even those who had maintained their weight.

Nuts and Bolts

Counting Calories
One pound equals 3500 calories. The average moderately active adult woman should consume 1800 to 2200 calories a day. If you cut 100 calories a day, you will lose one pound every 35 days. Likewise, if you add just 100 calories a day—about a third of a Snickers bar—you will add a pound every 35 days.

Diet: Healthy In, Healthy Out

In 1994, 2,437 women enrolled in a clinical trial to determine the effects of diet on breast cancer recurrence. All were postmenopausal and had been treated for early-stage breast cancer. Part of the women were given the support of dietitians who helped them maintain a healthy low-fat diet, with about 32 grams of fat a day. The others stayed on their normal diet of about 57 daily fat grams.

Researchers followed the women, ages 48 to 79, until 2001 and were pleased that the low-fat group consistently lost weight—an average of six pounds more than the regular diet group.[12]

The effects on breast cancer, though, surprised the scientists and many in the research community. The study showed a significant difference in how hormone-receptor-negative breast cancer related to diet. Women with estrogen-negative cancer who maintained the low-fat diet reduced their risk of recurrence by 42 percent more than the women not on the low-fat diet. Hormone-receptor-positive women had a 15 percent reduction.

Doctors expected the opposite result: Because fat intake can increase estrogen, they expected women with hormone-positive to have the greatest risk reduction. Researchers said this study, published in the *Journal of the National Cancer Institute* (2006), opened new avenues for follow-up breast cancer treatment.

BOX 6–3   **Is it low-fat or weight loss or?...**

Researchers and healthcare practitioners know that a plant-based diet is good for our overall health. They are less convinced that a low-fat diet by itself is the key to a reduced risk of triple-negative breast cancer.

A diet rich in fruits, vegetables, whole grains, beans, nuts, and seeds is naturally low in dietary fat and usually leads to weight loss. And this diet is linked to a reduction in our risk of a host of diseases, including type II diabetes, heart disease, breast and other forms of cancer, and arthritis.

So reducing fat is good for us in a multitude of ways. But is it the magic bullet that reduces the risk of TNBC? Not likely.

Participants in the Women's Intervention Nutrition Study (WINS) who reduced their dietary fat ultimately reduced their risk of hormone-negative cancer recurrence—but they also lost weight. At this point, it is unclear if their risk of recurrence was reduced specifically because of the low-fat diet or because of the weight loss that diet brought or by a combination of factors.

This study played an important role in my recovery for several reasons. It was the first full research report I read after I was diagnosed, and it provided significant hope. It showed that the approach I was taking to my health, which included eating well, had a payoff beyond my waistline. And it piqued my interest to see what else was out there about this disease that had taken up residence in my body. Cancer was a small part of my body, an unhealthy batch of cells out to do no good. The rest of me, though, was ready to do battle with my cellular invaders.

So this dietary research, part of the Women's Intervention Nutrition Study (WINS), offered just what I needed: a guide for taking care of my entire body that also might help me fight my specific brand of breast cancer. It's one of a host of studies that look at how everything from cantaloupe to cauliflower may be influenced by receptor status.

The WINS research was an initial toe dip into the pool of research on diet and hormone-negative cancer, and subsequent studies have challenged some of its findings while supporting others, as we will discuss later in this chapter. It was groundbreaking, though, in showing a connection between hormone-negative cancers and nutrition.

Nuts and Bolts

Five Ways to Maintain a Healthy Weight

Successful weight control means changing the way you live your life—the way you eat and your level of physical activity. And this is not a short-term thing. It is forever.

So don't diet. Dieting implies a temporary change built on forcing yourself to eat unnaturally. A boiled egg for breakfast, yogurt for lunch, salad for dinner. Nobody can sustain that, especially if you are fighting cancer or recuperating from treatment. And even if you conscientiously stick to the diet plan, you face trouble when you return to "normal" eating, which was what caused the weight gain to begin with.

Losing weight comes from changing your attitude toward food, seeing it as a source of energy and health, not a reward or a way to kill time. And eating healthy doesn't mean you've ruined the important social aspects of food. You can enjoy a convivial visit with friends over a well-balanced meal. Eating nutritious foods can be every bit as satisfying as eating the fatty stuff.

Remember that the pleasures of overeating are fleeting, but the results are long-lasting.

It takes a plan, though.

1. Be reasonable. If you've just been diagnosed, you need to think about treatment decisions, getting enough rest, and proper nutrition. So wait until treatment is over, and then bite off a small challenge. I started with a plan to lose 20 pounds, but the process became a part of my life and I kept at it until 50 pounds dropped. Had I started by saying I planned to lose 50, I likely would have been overwhelmed, impatient, and easily discouraged.

2. Write it down. Make a list of everything you eat, including calories, fats, and sugars. You'll be surprised at how much the little things add up. For example, a Snickers bar has 271 calories, 122 of those from fat. One bar has 26 percent of your daily recommended allotment of trans fat. It has a substantial 28.8 grams of sugar. So think about it: Look at the fleeting pleasure, the lasting damage. Numerous online sites can help you find nutrition information on the foods you eat.

3. Measure. If you have a glass of wine, look at the size. Five ounces of red wine has roughly 147 calories. Yet, do you limit yourself to that small a portion? Wine glasses often contain eight ounces, and we tend to fill them up, which raises the calorie count to 235. The larger glass, then, has 88 more calories. In 40 days, that extra wine will turn into a pound of fat. That's nine pounds a year. And research suggests keeping liquor consumption under one serving a day, which means less than five ounces.

4. Keep healthy snacks on hand. Don't let high-fat diet-busters even enter your house. If they are there, you will eat them. Do stock up on low-fat, nutritional goodies such as apples and other easy-to-nibble fruit, baby carrots, reduced-fat cheese, high-fiber cereal, and, my favorite, seeds and nuts.

5. Eat at home. Restaurants are full of temptations, and there's a reason they taste so good. Wonder why the pasta is so much better at your favorite Italian bistro than at home? Butter. Lots of it. An Alfredo dish—the kind that tastes really, really good—can contain up to 1500 calories and enough pasta for a family a four. Even a seemingly healthy side dish like sautéed spinach can be slathered in butter.

Food as a Health Tonic

When you think about it, it makes sense that the toxins we ingest will turn toxic in our bodies. We don't think about that, though, when we're faced with a golden batch of French fries or a creamy chocolate malt. At least, I didn't. My precancer diet was an embarrassment, and even after I went on my weight-loss regimen, I often focused on increasing my exercise to allow myself to eat far too badly.

I knew the healthy effects of a good diet; I just chose to generally ignore that knowledge. Cancer made me pay attention. I now look at fried foods and see a big batch of carcinogens. When I enjoy a salad of dark, leafy greens, I feel like I have just given my body a health tonic. When you look at the studies below, you'll see why.

A good diet does not ensure that you will beat your cancer or keep it from returning. It can, however, be an important element in keeping your overall body strong enough to fight, both physically and psychologically.

Healthy overall diet: Women who scored high on Harvard University's Alternate Healthy Eating Index had a lower risk of estrogen-negative breast cancer than those with a more common Western diet. The guidelines for this index: a daily intake of nine servings of fruits and veggies, seven or more grams of dietary fiber, 30 to 40 percent less saturated fat than polyunsaturated fats, fewer than 3 grams of trans fats, and 1 ounce of nuts.[13]

Antioxidants: Antioxidants are vitamins, minerals, and enzymes that help our bodies fight diseases such as cancer. They include vitamin C, vitamin E, and beta carotene (which turns into vitamin A in the body) and are found in everything from blueberries to melatonin. There is evidence that they can help fight breast cancer, although studies do not always differentiate between different receptor types.

An observational study of postmenopausal women, as part of the Women's Health Initiative and published in the *American Journal of Clinical Nutrition* (2008), found that both hormone-negative and hormone-positive breast cancer was reduced with vitamin C intake. Participants were given a daily average of 106 mg from diet and 350 mg from supplements.

And a study in *Journal of Investigative Medicine* (2009) of 49 women with breast cancer found that all showed DNA damage related to oxidation, which is the process antioxidants fight.[14] Risk of recurrence was reduced for postmenopausal women who took vitamin C and vitamin E supplements for more than three years, according to a *Journal of the National Cancer Institute* (2003) study.[15] And an *International Journal of Cancer* (2001) study showed that ascorbic acid—vitamin C—can benefit overweight women but offers limited help to women with a body mass index (BMI) under 25.[16]

Melatonin is a natural hormone that also acts as an antioxidant. The body produces it as part of a normal circadian rhythm regulated by light during the day and dark at night. A break in this cycle has shown connection to breast cancer. In research using Nurses Health Study data, women were found to be more at risk of breast cancer the longer they worked at night. This risk, however, was limited to hormone-positive and not hormone-negative breast cancer.[17]

In initial research on tumor cells at the City of Hope Beckman Research Institute, blueberry juice inhibited the growth of triple-negative breast cancer and slowed its spread.

Multivitamins: Studies on the effects of multivitamins have been all over the place, showing everything from significant effect to no effect at all. Some even indicate that multivitamins can increase cancer risk. If you have a balanced diet, though, with enough vitamins and minerals, you should need no multivitamins. Multivitamins can be a crutch, offering the illusion of doing something healthy. And one reason studies are so contradictory may be that they do not take into account the other things people do to keep their bodies healthy. It might be that a person with a healthy diet also takes a multivitamin; the reduced cancer risk might be from that diet and not the pill. Likewise, if the pills are used instead of a healthy diet, they offer no benefit.

BOX 6–4 **Can You Take Too Many Vitamins?**

Fat-soluble supplements are more of a problem than water-soluble. A meta-analysis of existing studies in *JAMA: The Journal of the American Medical Association* (2007) determined that overdoses of beta carotene, vitamin A, and vitamin E—all fat-soluble—can make you sick, with extreme cases being fatal. The risks of overdose of vitamin C, which is water-soluble, were not clear-cut and needed more study.[a]

Fat-soluble: These include beta-carotene and vitamins A, D, E, and K, which are stored in body fat tissues. Too many of these can build up in the liver, brain, and heart and may be toxic. Dangerous levels, though, are typically many times the suggested normal dose.

Water-soluble: B-complex and vitamin C are water-soluble, which means excess amounts are eliminated from

BOX 6–4   (Continued)

the body in the urine, which makes them less dangerous. Too much vitamin C can upset your stomach, though.

Natural sources: Your best bet for vitamins is to get them from vegetables, fruits, fish oils, low-fat dairy products, nuts, seeds, and whole grains. You're far less likely to overdose on carrots than on beta-carotene.

[a]Bjelakovic, Goran, Nikolova, Dimitrinka, Gluud, Lise L., Simonetti, Rosa G., and Gluud, Christian, "Mortality in randomized trials of antioxidant supplements for primary and secondary prevention: systematic review and meta-analysis," *JAMA*, vol. 297, no. 8, 842–857 (2007). Find the full article at http://jama.ama-assn.org/content/297/8/842.full.

Fruits and vegetables: Multiple studies have provided evidence that vegetables and fruits are natural cancer-fighters—and they are especially potent against hormone-negative breast cancer.

One study in *Nutritional Epidemiology* (2006) was designed specifically to gauge the association between receptor status and a healthy diet. Its most compelling finding: One serving of vegetables a day was associated with a 6 percent reduction in estrogen-negative cancer in postmenopausal women; each serving of fruit came with a 12 percent reduction.[18] Using data from the Nurses Health Study, researchers surveyed the eating habits of 3,580 postmenopausal women with breast cancer; 2,367 were estrogen-positive, 575 were estrogen-negative, and 838 cases could not be classified. All were given a variety of diets. The overall diet that showed the best results in reducing the risk of estrogen-negative breast cancer was high in vegetables, fruits, and whole grains, with low saturated fat and low-fat dairy products.

The Women's Healthy Eating and Living (WHEL) randomized trial also showed a significant benefit to regular servings daily of fruits and vegetables—in this case, five a day.[19] The WHEL study, published in *Journal of the American Medical Association* (2007), included more than 3,000 pre- and postmenopausal women, ages 18 to 70 years old, who were followed for seven years. Half the participants were given access to telephone counseling, cooking classes, and newsletters that promoted a daily diet of eight servings of fruits and vegetables—five vegetable, three fruit—plus 16 ounces of vegetable juice and an overall low-fat, high-fiber diet. A comparison group was asked to eat at least five fruit and vegetable servings per day.

Surprisingly, the enriched diet of eight servings was not the winner. Women in the comparison group, with five servings, who were also physically active, had nearly a 50 percent reduction in mortality, compared to women who had fewer servings and were less active. Eating even more vegetables and fruit showed no additional benefit. The results appeared consistent for all hormone receptor groups.

Cruciferous vegetables: A diet rich in cruciferous, or brassica, vegetables—like kale, cabbage, broccoli, bok choy, radishes, and cauliflower—can be effective in fighting triple-negative, according to a laboratory study published in *Breast Cancer Research* (2011). Researchers injected indole-3-carbinole (I3C), which occurs in high quantities in these vegetables, into cancer cells and found that it showed promise as an anticancer agent for TNBC tumors as well as for those that are hormone-positive.[20]

I3C showed success fighting cancer in earlier studies. Researchers from the University of California-Berkeley and the Kochi Medical School in Japan say it shows potential for combating the development of breast cancer cells.[21] Scientists in Italy came to much the same conclusion, using synthetic I3C.[22] While I3C tablets are commercially available, including cruciferous vegetables in your diet is a far healthier option.

Carbohydrates: Too many processed carbohydrates—sugar, white bread, cakes, and cookies—can increase a woman's risk of hormone-negative breast cancer, according to research in France published in *American Journal of Clinical Nutrition* (2008).[23] In the study, the dietary intake of 62,739 postmenopausal women was monitored from 1993 to 2002. Of these women, 1,812 eventually were diagnosed with breast cancer. Women who were overweight and had a large waist circumference were most at risk of breast cancer if their diet was high in processed carbs; cases of hormone-negative were directly associated with these carbs. The researchers speculate that because simple carbs are rapidly absorbed by the body, they elevate insulin levels, which may be the link to hormone-negative breast cancer.

And Swedish researchers monitored the diets of 15,773 women for slightly more than 10 years; in that time, 544 of the women were diagnosed with breast cancer. Researchers discovered that those who regularly consumed high-fiber bread had a significantly reduced risk of breast cancer—both hormone-negative and hormone-positive. Fried potatoes were significantly associated with an increase in hormone-negative breast cancer.[24] This does not mean that potatoes are specifically bad, just their fried form.

Don't confuse unhealthy processed carbs with their healthier cousins, complex carbohydrates—whole grains, seeds, vegetables, and most fruits. Complex carbs are more slowly digested and less likely to increase insulin levels. So switch to whole-grain breads, cereals, and pastas—look for the word "whole." Watch out for traps such as "multigrain," which sounds healthy but can simply mean a variety of processed carbs that are no better for you than plain white bread.

BOX 6–5   **Understanding Research**

Why do so many studies contradict one another? The promising results found in one trial might be completely discounted by another trial a year later. Which study is "right"? That's a difficult question to answer, as no two studies are alike, unless one is intended to replicate—duplicate—another as a means of testing the results, perhaps with added variables.

So how do you, as a consumer, make sense of this?

Look at the study population—age, type of cancer, tumor characteristics, and so on. Hormone receptor status can add an additional layer of difficulty, often because the sample size may be too small to draw adequate conclusions. Because fewer women are diagnosed with this disease—about 20 percent of all cancers are triple-negative—the sample size of the women in any study may be too small to be significant. And, on occasion, the connection to hormone receptors is not part of the original study design, so researchers make conclusions after the fact, rather than specifically studying those effects.

(Continued)

BOX 6–5 (Continued)

And pay attention to the type of study:

Clinical trials: Researchers test treatments or options—scientists call them *interventions*—such as surgery, drugs, radiation, diet, or physical activity on human subjects. The research consists of a study group, which is given the drug or treatment, and the placebo or control group, which does not receive treatment. The WINS and WHEL studies were both clinical trials. Initial clinical trials are phase I; success in these leads to phase II studies; and success there leads to the final study, or phase III. Successful phase III studies can lead to new drugs and treatment protocols.

Observational studies: Researchers observe a specific population through surveys, regular monitoring, and other tests, looking at how often a disease occurs in the study population, what the risk factors for a disease may be, what variables might be connected to the disease (weight gain, diet, specific chemotherapy treatments), or what the outcome of contracting a disease may be. Observational studies can include prospective cohort studies, which select groups with similar characteristics and follow them over time, to see how different variables affect them. The Nurses Health Study is a cohort study.

Laboratory studies: Scientists study cancer activity in test tubes or in animals. If their research is successful, it can ultimately lead to clinical trials in humans. These studies often use the term *in vitro*, meaning "in glass," referring to the test tube.

Meta-analysis: Researchers look at existing studies and combine that data to create a single "pool" of information for statistical analyses. Several of the vitamin D studies we discuss are meta-analyses, also called research reviews.

Fats: As we saw in the Women's Intervention Nutrition Study (WINS), a low-fat diet can be a vital cancer fighter. However, the Women's Healthy Eating and Living (WHEL) research came to a different conclusion, finding that reducing dietary fat intake did not reduce risk of recurrence or death. So what do we make of these competing results? One reason for the discrepancy between the WINS and the WHEL research is that they studied two significantly different groups of women. The WINS participants were all postmenopausal, while those in the WHEL study were both pre- and postmenopausal. The WHEL women did not undergo chemotherapy. In the WINS research, all hormone-negative participants received chemo; it was optional for hormone-positive patients.

Dissecting the two studies, we can come to two conclusions: First, postmenopausal women may need to watch their diet, including fat intake, more than premenopausal, an effect we saw in the Nurses

---

BOX 6–6   **The Skinny on Fats**

Not all fats are created equal, so it's important to pay attention to the type you include in your diet:

- Saturated fats are found in food that comes from animals—lard, butter, cheese, meat, poultry—and from tropical plants—coconut and palm oils. Avoid these as much as possible.
- Trans fats are made by a chemical process of hydrogenation of oils that increases the shelf life and the flavors of foods. Trans fat is found in vegetable shortenings and in some margarines, plus treats like packaged cookies, fries, and chips. Avoid them, period. New York City and the state of California ban them from their restaurants.
- Monounsaturated fats are "good" fats and are found in olive oil, canola oil, nuts, and avocados.
- Polyunsaturated fats are also "good." They include omega-3 fats (seafood, such as salmon, tuna, sardines,

(Continued)

> **BOX 6–6 (Continued)**
>
> mackerel, or shellfish, plus walnuts, flaxseed, and canola and soybean oils) and omega-6 fats (soybean, safflower, sunflower, or corn oils, nuts, and seeds).
>
> Your body needs some unsaturated fats to function so, in general, replace your saturated fats with mono- and polyunsaturated but don't go overboard. Good fats can still pack on the calories.

Health Study. And second, chemotherapy reduces the risk of recurrence for hormone-negative patients more than for hormone-positive; therefore, these women are more likely to respond to the benefits of a healthy diet because chemotherapy has already reduced their risks.

Caffeine: The more caffeine you consume, the higher your risk of hormone-negative breast cancer, according to research as part of the Women's Health Study, published in *Archives of Internal Medicine* (2008). Based on the responses of 39,310 participants who filled out a comprehensive questionnaire on their eating habits, the study looked at the links between caffeine intake—coffee, black tea, and colas primarily—and breast cancer.[25]

Researchers assumed that the content of caffeine was 137 mg per cup of coffee, 47 mg per cup of tea, 46 mg per can or bottle of cola, and 7 mg per serving of chocolate candy. The big caffeine killer here, then, is coffee.

Twenty-four percent of the women never drank coffee; 13 percent drank less than a cup a day; 14.2 percent had two to three cups a day, and 15.4 percent had four cups a day.

The risk of hormone-negative went up with each cup of coffee, as did the chance of having a tumor larger than 2 centimeters. No matter the quantity, though, caffeine had no significant effect on hormone-positive breast cancer.

However, the number of cases of hormone-negative breast cancer was so small that researchers noted that they didn't have enough data to state conclusively that high caffeine leads to hormone-negative breast cancer.

Research from Sweden's Karolinska Institute tells a different story, showing a connection between significant caffeine intake—more than five cups of coffee a day—and a reduction of risk in hormone-negative breast cancer.[26] The study focused on 6,000 postmenopausal women, who saw a 57 percent reduced risk of recurrence, whether or not they used hormone-replacement therapy or alcohol, and independent of their educational status. Researchers suggest that compounds in coffee, such as trigonelline, may provide some level of protection. Hormone-receptor status was available for only 65 percent of those studied, however. Some things to remember: This research involved postmenopausal women, and TNBC is more likely to affect premenopausal women, so the effects on that population are not clear. Likewise, other dietary effects may come into play here—it could be that these women had a healthier overall diet or a healthier lifestyle otherwise, so the effects of caffeine were mediated by other factors. In addition, the types of coffee they drank may have been specific to Sweden and not to other countries.

The bottom line is that too much caffeine in general is not good for you. And who needs the extra nervousness that coffee brings when you are already stressed?

Vitamin D: Studies of the benefits of vitamin D may seem inconsistent, with some showing significant benefits and others showing none, and most not differentiating between hormone receptor types. The difference often is in the study design. Studies on serum vitamin D—the form that circulates in the blood—often find more cancer-fighting evidence. Those that study vitamin D intake are less convincing. This could be because our bodies use vitamin D differently, depending on a variety of factors: age, diet, activity level, and even genetics. Also, serum vitamin D comes from the most natural of all sources—the sun or our diets—whereas vitamin D intake studies often measure artificial forms. Still, even researchers who study the serum form advocate having your vitamin D levels tested and taking supplements as needed, especially for people in northern latitudes who do not have the benefit of regular sunny days.

A case study of 91 breast cancer patients in Whittier, California, found that those with triple-negative were more likely to be deficient in serum vitamin D—a form called 25 (OH)D. Fifteen of the patients were triple-negative, and the majority of those—87 percent—had lower levels of the vitamin than other cancer patients, with the remaining 13 percent being borderline. This was a small, but in-depth study.[27]

A specific form of active vitamin D3 known as Gemini 0097 substantially reduced the development of both estrogen-negative and estrogen-positive breast cancer on rats, according to lab research done at Rutgers University and published in *Cancer Prevention Research* (2008). Scientists injected rats with breast cancers then treated them with Gemini 0097. The vitamin D slowed the growth of estrogen-positive by 60 percent and estrogen-negative by 50 percent. Researchers note that Gemini 0097 is less toxic than other forms of synthetic vitamin D and does not lead to an overload of calcium, the vitamin's most common side effect.[28]

Several research reviews—also called meta-analyses—support the benefits of vitamin D. According to an *Annals of Epidemiology* (2009) review done by scientists at the University of California, San Diego, low levels of serum Vitamin D are connected to a variety of cancers, including breast, colon, ovarian, renal, pancreatic, and aggressive forms of prostate. Researchers projected that raising our intake of vitamin D would prevent 58,000 new cases of breast cancer each year; 2000 mg a day, they say, can increase serum levels to a healthier range without other risks.[29]

In a *Cancer Epidemiology, Biomarkers & Prevention* (2006) review, scientists cited numerous studies that link both calcium and vitamin D to reduced breast cancer risk for premenopausal as well as postmenopausal women.[30] And in another review, in *Annals of Epidemiology* (2007), researchers noted that 2000 IU a day of vitamin D3 can reduce the risk of breast cancer by 50 percent.[31]

Research on 16,818 participants in the Third National Health and Nutrition Examination Survey (NHANES III) determined that women with higher levels of serum vitamin D (over 25 ng/mL) had only about one-fourth the mortality rate from breast cancer as those with lower amounts. Survey participants were 17 years or older at enrollment and were followed from 1988 through 2000. The research was published in *Journal of the National Cancer Institute* (2007).[32]

Yet a long-term study—seven years—of postmenopausal women as part of the Women's Health Initiative and published in *Journal of the National Cancer Institute* (2008) found no relationship between vitamin D and breast cancer. Researchers gave women 1000 mg of elemental calcium with 400 IUs of vitamin D3 daily. Those women had no lower risk of breast cancer than those receiving a placebo.[33]

And research using data from the Cancer Prevention Study-II Nutrition Study also found no association between postmenopausal breast cancer risk and levels of vitamin D, regardless of hormone receptor status, body mass index, postmenopausal hormone therapy, weight gain, season of the year, or calcium intake.[34] However, researchers did note that the source of vitamin D might be important, with women who get the vitamin through their diet—in fortified milk or fish, for example—having higher levels circulating in their bodies. Also, dietary vitamin D is strongly correlated with calcium, which may be effective in fighting breast cancer. In addition, women living at northern latitudes get less vitamin D from the sun and are more likely to have breast cancer than those in southern latitudes.

BOX 6–7   **Sources of Vitamin D**

Natural sources of vitamin D are more effective than supplements, with the best source being UV rays from the sun. According to the National Institutes of Health, researchers recommend five to 30 minutes of sun exposure to the face, arms, legs, or back, without sunscreen, from 10 a.m. to 3 p.m. at least twice a week.[a] However, those of us in sun-challenged areas of the country—a line above 42 degrees latitude, or roughly above the northern border of California and Boston—don't get enough sun between November and February. Smog, shade, and cloud cover all reduce the sun's effectiveness elsewhere. And UV rays cannot penetrate glass, so sitting in front of a window may feel good, but it offers little vitamin D benefit.

But where do we get vitamin D if not from the sun? Some of the best sources:

Cod liver oil (1 tablespoon): 1360 IU
Sockeye salmon (3 ounces): 794 IU
Vitamin D-fortified milk (1 cup): 115–124 IU
Vitamin D-fortified orange juice (1 cup): 100 IU
One egg yolk: 25 IU

If you cannot get enough natural vitamin D, go for supplements. Studies show that vitamin D3 is as much as three

(Continued)

BOX 6–7   **(Continued)**

times as effective as other forms of vitamin D.[b] The National Institutes of Health recommend 600–800 IUs daily, although some research indicates that this amount can be safely increased, up to 2,000 IUs. Initial research has tied excessive amounts of vitamin D—over 2,000 IUs—to skin cancer.

[a]"Dietary supplement fact sheet: vitamin D," National Institutes of Health Office of Dietary Supplements, http://dietary-supplements.info.nih.gov/factsheets/vitamind.asp#en27 (accessed online December 2, 2009).
[b]Cranney, A., Horsley, T., O'Donnell, S., Weiler, H., Puil, L., Ooi, D., Atkinson, S., Ward, L., Moher, D., Hanley, D., Fang, M., Yazdi, F., Garritty, C., Sampson, M., Barrowman, N., Tsertsvadze, A., and Mamaladze, V., "Effectiveness and safety of vitamin D in relation to bone health" *Evidence Report-Technology Assessment*, no. 158, 1–235 (2007).

Alcohol: The effects of alcohol on breast cancer have been studied for decades, with varied results. Several studies have linked alcohol to breast cancer, most notably associating a family history of breast cancer, alcohol consumption, and hormone-negative disease.[35] Others have found less of a risk, or have found the risk limited to hormone-positive breast cancer.[36,37] A 2008 study categories the risk, which again is limited to hormone-positive, showing that one drink a day of alcohol of any type—beer, wine, spirits—increased breast cancer risk by 10 percent. The risk rose by the drink—three daily drinks equaled a 30 percent risk.[38] This is a relative risk—it is compared to the risk faced by a woman who drinks no alcohol or less than one drink a day. Rather than trying to decipher the studies, a healthy approach is to limit alcohol to an average of less than one drink a day, even if the research is not definitive in terms of hormone receptor status.

Alcohol and hormone replacement therapy: It may not be alcohol alone that increases the risk of breast cancer—it could be hormone replacement therapy (HRT) plus alcohol. According to Danish research published in the *International Journal of Cancer* (2008), postmenopausal women taking oral estrogen who had one or two alcoholic drinks a day increased their breast cancer risk by three times that of women who neither drank nor took HRT. Those who took HRT and had more than two drinks a day increased their risk to five times that of those who ingested neither HRT nor alcohol.[39] The research did not narrow its findings by receptor status, but HRT is more strongly associated with hormone-positive than with hormone-negative disease.

Folic acid: Folic acid is the synthetic form of the B vitamin folate, which helps form our DNA, which is why a diet rich in folate is

---

BOX 6–8   **Smoking and Hormone-Negative**

Smoking has been associated with multiple cancers, specifically lung, but also of the throat, mouth, pancreas, kidney, bladder, and cervix. And there is some evidence that smoking—even for those who gave up the habit—is associated with an increased risk of hormone-negative breast cancer. In a long-term study, 10,902 women, 35 percent of whom were smokers, were followed for an average of 12.4 years. Those who smoked had an increased risk of hormone-negative breast cancer, but not of hormone-positive. Ex-smokers specifically had an increased risk of progesterone-negative breast cancer.[a]

However, postmenopausal women who smoke do not face an increased risk of TNBC, according to research using data from the Women's Health Initiative. The study enrolled 148,030 women, 300 of whom had TNBC and 2,479 of whom had estrogen-positive disease. Smoking and alcohol use were both associated with ER-positive breast cancer, but not with TNBC. The research was published in *Cancer Causes Control* (2011).[b]

[a]Manjer, J., Malina, J., Berglund, G., Bondeson, L., Garne, J. P., and Janzon, L., "Smoking associated with hormone receptor negative breast cancer," *International Journal of Cancer*, vol. 91, no. 4, 580–584 (2001).
[b]Kabat, Geoffrey C., Kim, Mimi, Phipps, Amanda I., Li, Christopher I., Messina, Catherine R., Wactawski-Wende, Jean, Kuller, Lewis, Simon, Michael S., Yasmeen, Shagufta, Wassertheil-Smoller, Sylvia, and Rohan, Thomas E., "Smoking and alcohol consumption in relation to risk of triple-negative breast cancer in a cohort of postmenopausal women," *Cancer Causes and Control: CCC*, pp. 1–9 (2011).

important in fighting cancer. Using data from the Nurses Health Study, researchers determined that high levels of folic acid may reduce the risk of breast cancer.[40] The importance of folic acid especially comes into play in its relationship with alcohol, which depletes the body's stores of folic acid—and that may be one reason it leads to an increased cancer risk. And just 600 micrograms of folic acid a day can reduce the effect of alcohol on breast cancer risk.[41]

Foods rich in folate include dark green leafy vegetables, beans and peas, citrus juice, and fortified cereals.

Fish oil: Triple-negative breast cancers that metastasize typically move to the lungs or liver, which is called visceral metastasis.[42] A clinical trial in England demonstrates that use of docosahexaenoic acid (DHA)—found in cold water fish, fatty fish, fish oil supplements, and seaweed—along with chemotherapy can extend life for these patients, with few side effects.[43]

The study, published in the *British Journal of Cancer* (2009), was a phase II clinical trial enrolling 25 breast cancer patients with visceral metastases at University Hospital in Bretonneau in Tours, France. Patients were given 1800 mg of DHA a day—nine total capsules, three at each meal. The patients started this regimen before chemotherapy and continued it throughout five months of chemo. The median age of participants was 58; 72 percent had liver metastases, and 40 percent had three or more metastatic sites.

Chemo consisted of FEC: cyclophosphamide and fluorouracil followed by an IV infusion of epirubicin administered every 3 weeks. (This is common in Europe but not in the United States.) DHA was suspended on the day of chemotherapy. Duration was at least six cycles.

Median overall survival was 22 months, with a high of 34 months.

Those with the longest survival had the highest DHA intake. Previous studies had shown overall survival rates for FEC of 18–23 months.[44]

Researchers suggest that DHA strengthens the noncancerous cells, giving them more oomph to fight against cancer.

Other research demonstrates that women with the BRCA1 gene can benefit from omega-3 fatty acids. The study, part of the Singapore Chinese Health Study, showed that omega-3s from fish and shellfish reduced the risk of breast cancer; patients who had the highest levels in their diets had a 26 percent reduced risk of breast cancer. Researchers found no relationship with omega-6 fatty acids. And, while only a small percentage of those studied had the BRCA1 gene, those benefited the most.[45]

Soy: Women with either estrogen-negative or estrogen-positive breast cancers benefit from high soy intake, according to research in China.[46] Results were based on data from the Shanghai Breast Cancer Survival Study, a large, population-based cohort study of 5,042 female breast cancer survivors, aged 20 to 75 years, diagnosed between March 2002 and April 2006. Women were interviewed about their diet at 18, 36, and 60 months after diagnosis. Those with the highest intake of soy had the lowest recurrence rates. No toxic effects of soy were discovered. Soy contains folate, fiber, and calcium, all of which have been shown to be beneficial in reducing cancer.

Soy, however, is controversial because of its ability to stimulate estrogen receptors. While that might not seem like an issue with hormone-negative disease, it still might be safest to limit intake and to focus on natural, fresh soy as a legume, such as in edamame, rather than processed soy products in the form of burgers, powders, or capsules. Especially avoid soy protein isolate, soy protein concentrate, hydrolyzed soy protein, and texturized soy protein. Or get your folate, fiber, and calcium from other sources: vegetables, whole grains, nuts, seeds, and dairy products.

Organic foods: To meet USDA standards, organic fruits and vegetables are grown without chemical pesticides, herbicides, fumigants, or synthetic fertilizers and have not been irradiated or genetically engineered or modified. Dairy products, meats, and poultry come from animals that have been given no antibiotics, hormones, or growth stimulants; they have access to the outdoors and have been fed with certified organic feed.

Organic foods may be important in a cancer-fighting diet specifically because of their lack of chemical pesticides and hormones. According to the Environmental Protection Agency, chemical pesticides have been linked to cancer.[47] And ingestion of synthetic hormones may affect the body's natural hormone system, which is an issue in all breast cancers.

Look for the USDA seal for proof that the food is truly organic. The Environmental Working Group (EWG) offers a list of fruits and vegetables with the most chemical pesticides. Their "Dirty Dozen," those with the most chemicals, are: peaches, apples, sweet bell peppers, celery, nectarines, strawberries, cherries, kale, lettuce, imported grapes, carrots, and pears.[48]

Putting It All Together

Looking at studies like these and hearing about additional research on the nightly news sends many women to the health food store for multiple supplements. Or to the pain relief aisle. The best approach for TNBC and other forms of hormone-negative, though, is to get your nutrients through your diet, exercise regularly, and maintain a healthy weight:

- Make sure you have at least five servings of vegetables and fruits a day, and make sure you include cruciferous veggies like kale, cabbage, and broccoli.
- Cut saturated and trans fats from your diet—fats found in fried foods, butter, and creams—and replace them with healthy mono- and polyunsaturated fats (omega-3 and omega-6) found in fish, avocados, and flaxseed. Use oil and vinegar on your salads, lemon oil on veggies, and olive or flax oil on your whole-grain bread.
- Take a fish oil supplement if you can't get enough omega-3s in your diet; aim for 450–500 mg per day of combined EPA/DHA, which are polyunsaturated fatty acids.
- Limit unhealthy carbohydrates—sugar, white flour, cakes, and other sweet goodies.
- Increase healthy carbs—whole grains, seeds, vegetables, and most fruits.
- Avoid fried foods, period.
- Reduce your alcohol intake to 3–4 drinks a week and your caffeine to the equivalent of less than one cup of coffee a day. Switch to decaffeinated coffee or tea.
- Get at least 1200 mg of calcium a day. At least half of this should come from diet, such as yogurt, milk, and cheese, so you should be fine with 600 mg daily in supplement form. Make sure you take a calcium supplement with magnesium, as this helps calcium enter the system and keeps it from causing constipation.

- Add extra vitamin D—2000 IU a day—if you are in a northern latitude. Get 20 minutes of sun a day when possible. Avoid overdosing, either on the sun or on pills.
- Exercise three to four hours a week. Moderate or vigorous is best, but do what you can.
- Aim for a BMI between 21 and 25.
- If you can afford them, buy organic dairy products, natural meats, and fruits and vegetables on the Environmental Working Group's Dirty Dozen list.
- Stop smoking. Even if the influence of smoking on TNBC is unclear, why risk other forms of cancer?

Nuts and Bolts

The Triple-Negative Diet

This is the approach I take, based on the research I have done. It works for me, but you have to find what works best for you. Choose an approach you know you can stick to. Don't try to be Super Healthy Cancer Woman—that just adds more stress. Aim to be as healthy as you can be, and allow yourself to fall off the wagon occasionally. That is the only way you will stay with this long-term.

Breakfast: According to the National Weight Control Registry at Brown University Medical School, 78 percent of the people who lost more than 30 pounds and kept it off for more than a year regularly ate breakfast.[49] I always eat breakfast; my two approaches to it:

- A breakfast smoothie with blueberries (antioxidants), flaxseeds (cancer-fighting fiber), bananas, black cherry (more antioxidants) juice, and yogurt (bone-building and cancer-fighting calcium). This gives me two servings of fruits and one serving of calcium. Make sure you use ground flaxseed, because whole seeds just go right through you. And once they are ground, store them in the refrigerator.
- Cooked oatmeal with blueberries. It's simple—just follow the directions for one serving on the oatmeal box, and add about

1/2 cup of blueberries. Oatmeal soaks up cholesterol, so it is good for your heart as well.

Mid-morning snack: A piece of fruit, 1/8 cup of seeds, and 6–8 almonds.

Lunch: Eat a hearty but healthy lunch—you should expend more calories here than at dinner. I opt for soups, salads, whole-wheat pasta dishes, or sandwiches with low-fat whole-wheat bread. I look for combinations of spinach, broccoli, asparagus, green beans, romaine, and other dark greens; low-fat cheeses or yogurt; and whole grains. Tuna or egg salad sandwiches made with low-fat mayonnaise or yogurt and low-fat whole-wheat bread; 1/2 fresh bell pepper sliced; and a spinach salad makes a nice little lunch. I often treat myself to a scoop of frozen yogurt for dessert. One scoop is enough to satisfy me. (Usually.)

Midday snack: Some of my favorites:

- Broccoli and cauliflower dipped in hummus.
- Whole-wheat crackers and organic low-fat cheese.
- Popcorn (a whole grain that folks tend to ignore) with a light covering of sea salt. No butter.
- Homemade trail mix of pumpkin seeds, sunflower seeds, raisins, unsweetened dried cranberries, and almonds. You need no extra salt or sugar.
- Strips of bell peppers, powerful antioxidants high in vitamin C and E. (Red peppers are especially nutrient-rich; a small one contains 46 percent of your daily requirement of vitamin A and 158 percent of your vitamin C. By contrast, a green pepper of the same size has 5 percent of your daily vitamin A and 99 percent of your vitamin C.)

Juiced veggies every evening: This includes three to four carrots, one to two leaves of kale, 1/8 cabbage, one bunch parsley, one stalk celery, 1/4 apple, and 1/4 lemon. My super-juicing husband uses an auger juicer that takes the pulp out and leaves only the juice. This gives me two to three servings of veggies and is heavy on cancer-fighting cruciferous vegetables—kale and cabbage. The lemon, apple, and celery really help the taste.

Dinner: I go mostly vegetarian, with some fish and seafood.

- I have come to love sushi made with avocados, eggs, cucumbers, and celery (I'm not ready to try raw fish).
- Menus planned around broiled or baked fish or meat are good; combine this with steamed vegetables, brown rice, or sweet potatoes.
- Stir-fry is an easy way to combine brown rice, shrimp or chicken, and veggies such as broccoli and bok choy. Avoid cheese sauces and gravy—these are delicious gutters of calories.
- Soup and salad is healthy and easy. A cup of tomato soup and a spinach salad with vinaigrette gives you a couple of servings of vegetables with minimal calories. Bean soup can be a great source of protein as well as vitamins and minerals.
- For dessert, consider angel food cake, frozen yogurt, or a few squares of dark chocolate, which, yes, is an antioxidant. Milk chocolate is not.

Profile

An Alternative Approach

Noreen Parks is a science and environmental writer, so she approached her diagnosis of triple-negative breast cancer more scientifically than most. With respect for both Western medicine and its alternatives, she wanted to choose the best route to combat the stage 1 cancer she was diagnosed with in September 2004. In the end, she chose to undergo surgery and partial breast irradiation, followed by a regimen of alternative therapies, including intravenous infusions of ascorbic acid (vitamin C).

She caught the cancer early, finding the tumor herself in a monthly breast exam. A few weeks after the diagnosis, she had a lumpectomy to remove the 1.2 × 1.7-centimeter tumor. When she woke up after the operation, her surgeon told her that she had clear margins and her lymph nodes were normal. "You are now cancer-free," he said. But in a postsurgery appointment, he also told her that her she had triple-negative breast cancer, which meant she had very limited options for follow-up therapy. He urged her to have chemotherapy, as did three oncologists she consulted.

But she was not convinced. "After all my reporting on the effects of toxic chemicals in the environment, the thought of pumping in a bunch of chemicals to kill cells—including my healthy ones— just didn't make sense to me. It felt contrary to my health philosophy," says Noreen, who was 55 at diagnosis. "Whatever course I decided to take, I knew I had to be 100 percent on board with it." In her case, with a small tumor that had not spread, she believed the survivorship statistics did not persuasively support chemotherapy. "It seemed like a gamble with a huge price to pay for a potentially small gain. And *none* of us is a statistic."

As she researched alternative treatment options, she learned about a relatively new type of breast irradiation: brachytherapy, or partial breast therapy. In contrast to whole breast external radiation, this approach uses the placement of tiny pellets of radioactive material inside an area that may contain residual cancer cells following surgery. "Since the vast majority of recurrent tumors occur very close to the site of the original one, this seemed like a smarter, safer way to deliver radiation," Noreen says. She underwent the recommended course of treatment—twice a day for five days in total—at a hospital in Hawaii, where she lived before moving to Washington.

Next, she met with a complementary and alternative medicine (CAM) doctor—previously a cardiologist—in Hawaii. His patients included women with breast cancer. "His approach was comprehensive, holistic, and focused on addressing factors that might have weakened my immune system and on fully restoring my health," she says. He mapped out a path of treatment and told her she could always do chemo later. To begin with, she went on a 90-day, low-carbohydrate, high-protein diet. "Sugar feeds cancer," her doctor frequently reminded her.

Her complete physical exam included a hair analysis for heavy metals, which showed that her body had elevated levels of lead, mercury, and cadmium—known carcinogens. She underwent intravenous chelation therapy to remove them. Then she took a series of intravenous ascorbic-acid infusions, a treatment pioneered decades ago by Nobel laureate Linus Pauling. She found scientists at the National Institutes of Health who were studying the use of ascorbic acid on cancer cells in lab tests with success.[50] She corresponded with the researchers for more detailed information and felt secure in her choice of what she calls "natural chemotherapy." A year later, she underwent a second round of six treatments, "for insurance," she says.

"Then I went on to live my life," she says. "I have always been physically active—swimming, hiking, kayaking, biking. I take vitamins and other supplements and watch my diet. Our refrigerator is loaded with fresh food, very little processed stuff. I don't eat red meat, but I eat some chicken and fish. 'Eat to live' is a maxim around our house."

Noreen celebrated her seven-year anniversary in 2011. Summing up her cancer experience, she says, "One of the toughest things about cancer is the initial feeling of helplessness. Asking lots of questions and learning as much as you can about breast cancer and your individual situation empowers you to make the right decisions for *you*. I think Western medicine has a lot to offer, but it does not have all the answers."

Notes

1. Check out Julie's blog at http://jadesloge.livejournal.com/#asset-jadesloge-28890.
2. Phipps, Amanda I., Chlebowski, Rowan T., Prentice, Ross, McTiernan, Anne, Stefanick, Marcia L., Wactawski-Wende, Jean, Kuller, Lewis H., Adams-Campbell, Lucile L., Lane, Dorothy, Vitolins, Mara, Kabat, Geoffrey C., Rohan, Thomas E., and Li, Christopher I., "Body size, physical activity, and risk of triple-negative and estrogen receptor-positive breast cancer," *Cancer Epidemiology, Biomarkers & Prevention*, vol. 20, no. 3, 454–463 (2011).
3. For more information on the various studies using data from the California Teachers Study, go to http://www.calteachersstudy.org/index.html.
4. Dallal, Cher M., Sullivan-Halley, Jane, Ross, Ronald K., Wang, Ying, Deapen, Dennis, Horn-Ross, Pamela L., Reynolds, Peggy, Stram, Daniel O., Clarke, Christina A., Anton-Culver, Hoda, Ziogas, Argyrios, Peel, David, West, Dee W., Wright, William, and Bernstein, Leslie, "Long-term recreational physical activity and risk of invasive and in situ breast cancer: the California Teachers

Study," *Archives of Internal Medicine*, vol. 167, no. 4, 408–415 (2007).

5. Enger, Shelley M., Ross, Ronald K., Paganini-Hill, Annlia, Carpenter, Catherine L., and Bernstein, Leslie, "Body size, physical activity, and breast cancer hormone receptor status: results from two case-control studies," *Cancer Epidemiology, Biomarkers & Prevention*, vol. 9, no. 7, 681–687 (2000).

6. Maruti, Sonia S., Willett, Walter C., Feskanich, Diane, Rosner, Bernard, and Colditz, Graham A., "A prospective study of age-specific physical activity and premenopausal breast cancer," *Journal of the National Cancer Institute*, vol. 100, no. 10, 728–737 (2008). Get a PDF at http://jnci.oxfordjournals.org/content/100/10/728.full.pdf.

7. Courneya, Kerry S., Katzmarzyk, Peter T., and Bacon, Eric, "Physical activity and obesity in Canadian cancer survivors," *Cancer*, vol. 112, no. 11, 2475–2482 (2008). Find the full article at http://onlinelibrary.wiley.com/doi/10.1002/cncr.23455/full.

8. Renehan, Andrew G., Tyson, Margaret, Egger, Matthias, Heller, Richard F., and Zwahlen, Marcel, "Body-mass index and incidence of cancer: a systematic review and meta-analysis of prospective observational studies," *Lancet*, vol. 371, no. 9612, 569–578 (2008).

9. Department of Health and Human Services, National Institute of Health, "Learn about body mass index," http://www.nhlbi.nih.gov/health/public/heart/obesity/wecan/learn-it/bmi-chart.htm (accessed June 11, 2009).

10. Nichols, Hazel B., Trentham-Dietz, Amy, Egan, Kathleen M., Titus-Ernstoff, Linda, Holmes, Michelle D., Bersch, Andrew J., Holick, Crystal N., Hampton, John M., Stampfer, Meir J., Willett, Walter C., and Newcomb, Polly A., "Body mass index before and after breast cancer diagnosis: associations with all-cause, breast cancer, and cardiovascular disease mortality," *Cancer Epidemiology, Biomarkers & Prevention*, vol. 18, no. 5, 1403–1409 (2000). Find the full article at http://cebp.aacrjournals.org/content/18/5/1403.full.pdf+html.

11. Eliassen, A. Heather, Colditz, Graham A., Rosner, Bernard, Willett, Walter C., and Hankinson, Susan E., "Adult weight change and risk of postmenopausal breast cancer," *Journal of the American Medical Association*, vol. 296, no. 2, 193–201 (2006). Find the

full article at http://jama.ama-assn.org/content/296/2/193.full.
pdf+html.

12. Chlebowski, Rowan T., Blackburn, George L., Thomson, Cynthia A., Nixon, Daniel W., Shapiro, Alice, Hoy, M. Katherine, Goodman, Marc T., Giuliano, Armando E., Karanja, Njeri, McAndrew, Philomena, Hudis, Clifford, Butler, John, Merkel, Douglas, Kristal, Alan, Caan, Bette, Michaelson, Richard, Vinciguerra, Vincent, Del Prete, Salvatore, Winkler, Marion, Hall, Rayna, Simon, Michael, Winters, Barbara L., and Elashoff, Robert M., "Dietary fat reduction and breast cancer outcome: interim efficacy results from the Women's Intervention Nutrition Study," *Journal of the National Cancer Institute.* vol. 98, no. 24,1767–1776 (2006). Find the full article at http://jnci.oxfordjournals.org/content/98/24/1767.full.
pdf+html.

13. Fung, Teresa T., Hu, Frank B., Barbieri, Robert L., Willett, Walter C., and Hankinson, Susan E., "Dietary patterns, the Alternate Healthy Eating Index and plasma sex hormone concentrations in postmenopausal women," *International Journal of Cancer*, vol. 121, no. 4, 803–809 (2007). Find a PDF at http://onlinelibrary.
wiley.com/doi/10.1002/ijc.22728/pdf.

14. Himmetoglu, Solen, Dincer, Yildiz, Ersoy, Yeliz E., Bayraktar, Baris, Celik, Varol, and Akcay, Tulay, "DNA oxidation and antioxidant status in breast cancer," *Journal of Investigative Medicine*, vol. 57, no. 6, 720–723 (2009).

15. Fleischauer, Aaron T., Simonsen, Neal, and Arab, Lenore, "Antioxidant supplements and risk of breast cancer recurrence and breast cancer-related mortality among postmenopausal women," *Nutrition and Cancer*, vol. 46, no. 1, 15–22 (2003).

16. Michels, K. B., Holmberg, L., Bergkvist, L., Ljung, H., Bruce, A., and Wolk, A., "Dietary antioxidant vitamins, retinol, and breast cancer incidence in a cohort of Swedish women," *International Journal of Cancer*, vol. 91, no. 4, 563–567 (2001).

17. Schernhammer, Eva S., Laden, Francine, Speizer, Frank E., Willett, Walter C., Hunter, David J., Kawachi, Ichiro, and Colditz, Graham A., "Rotating night shifts and risk of breast cancer in women participating in the Nurses' Health Study," *Journal of the National Cancer Institute*, vol. 93, no. 20, 1563–1568 (2001). Find the full article at http://jnci.oxfordjournals.org/cgi/content/full/93/20/156 3?ijkey=co1d8ce29cboba35061db9c434a0c8e4816e70a9.

18. Fung, Teresa T., Hu, Frank B., McCullough, Marjorie L., Newby, P. K.,Willett, Walter C., and Holmes, Michelle D., "Diet quality is associated with the risk of estrogen receptor–negative breast cancer in postmenopausal women," *Nutritional Epidemiology*, vol. 136, no. 2, 466–472 (2006). Find the full article at http://jn.nutrition.org/cgi/reprint/136/2/466.pdf.

19. Pierce, John P., Natarajan, Loki, Caan, Bette J., Parker, Barbara A., Greenberg, E. Robert, Flatt, Shirley W., Rock, Kealey, Cheryl L., Al-Delaimy, Sheila, Bardwell, Wael K., Carlson, Wayne A., Emond, Robert W., Faerber, Jennifer A., Gold, Susan, Hajek, Ellen, Hollenbach, Richard A., Jones, Kathryn, Karanja, Lovell A., Madlensky, Njeri, Marshall, Lisa, Newman, James, Ritenbaugh, Vicky A., Thomson, Cheryl, Wasserman, Linda, and Stefanick, Marcia L., "Influence of a diet very high in vegetables, fruit, and fiber and low in fat on prognosis following treatment for breast cancer: the Women's Healthy Eating and Living (WHEL) randomized trial," *JAMA: The Journal of the American Medical Association*, vol. 298, no. 3, 289–298 (2007). Find the full article at http://jama.ama-assn.org/cgi/content/full/298/3/289.

20. De Santi, Mauro, Galluzzi, Luca, Lucarini, Simone, Paoletti, Maria F., Fraternale, Alessandra, Duranti, Andrea, De Marco, Cinzia, Fanelli, Mirco, Zaffaroni, Nadia, Brandi, Giorgio, and Magnani, Mauro, "The indole-3-carbinol cyclic tetrameric derivative CTet inhibits cell proliferation via overexpression of p21/CDKN1A in both estrogen receptor positive and triple negative breast cancer cell lines," *Breast Cancer Research*, vol. 13, no. 2, R33+ (2011).

21. Chatterji, Urmi, Riby, Jacques E., Taniguchi, Taketoshi, Bjeldanes, Erik L., Bjeldanes, Leonard F., and Firestone, Gary L., "Indole-3-carbinol stimulates transcription of the interferon gamma receptor 1 gene and augments interferon responsiveness in human breast cancer cells," *Carcinogenesis*, vol. 25, no. 7, 1119–1128 (2004).

22. Brandi, Giorgio, Paiardini, Mirko, Cervasi, Barbara, Fiorucci, Chiara, Filippone, Paolino, De Marco, Cinzia, Zaffaroni, Nadia, and Magnani, Mauro, "A new indole-3-carbinol tetrameric derivative inhibits cyclin-dependent kinase 6 expression, and induces G1 cell cycle arrest in both estrogen-dependent and estrogen-independent breast cancer cell lines," *Cancer Research*, vol. 63,

no. 14, 4028–4036 (2003). Find the full article at http://cancerres. aacrjournals.org/content/63/14/4028.full.pdf+html.

23. Lajous, Martin, Boutron-Ruault, Marie-Christine, Fabre, Alban, Clavel-Chapelon, Francoise, and Romieu, Isabelle, "Carbohydrate intake, glycemic index, glycemic load, and risk of postmeno-pausal breast cancer in a prospective study of French women," *American Journal of Clinical Nutrition*, vol. 87, no. 5, 1384–1391 (2008). Find the full article at http://www.ajcn.org/cgi/content/ full/87/5/1384.

24. Sonestedt, E., Borgquist, S., Ericson, U., Gullberg, B., Landberg, G., Olsson, H., and Wirfält, E., "Plant foods and oestrogen recep-tor α- and β defined breast cancer: observations from the Malmö Diet and Cancer cohort," *Carcinogenesis*, vol. 29, no. 11, 2203–2209 (2008). Find the full article at http://carcin.oxfordjournals. org/content/29/11/2203.full.pdf+html.

25. Ishitani, Ken, Lin, Jennifer, Manson, JoAnn E., Buring, Julie E., and Zhang, Shumin M., "Caffeine consumption and the risk of breast cancer in a large prospective cohort of women," *Archives of Internal Medicine*, vol. 168, no. 18, 2022–2031 (2008). Find the full article at http://archinte.ama-assn.org/cgi/content/ abstract/168/18/2022.

26. Li, Jingmei, Seibold, Petra, Claude, Jenny C., Janys, Dieter F., Liu, Jianjun, Czene, Kamila, Humphreys, Keith, and Hall, Per, "Coffee consumption modifies risk of estrogen-receptor negative breast cancer," *Breast Cancer Research*, vol. 13, no. 3, R49+ (2011). Find the full article at http://breast-cancer-research.com/content/pdf/ bcr2879.pdf.

27. Rainville, Christa, Khan, Yasir Tisman, Glenn, "Triple negative breast cancer patients presenting with low serum vitamin D lev-els: a case series," *Cases Journal*, vol. 2 (2009), http://www.ncbi. nlm.nih.gov:80/pmc/articles/PMC2740106/.

28. Lee, Hong Jin J., Paul, Shiby, Atalla, Nadi, Thomas, Paul E., Lin, Xinjie, Yang, Ill, Buckley, Brian, Lu, Gang, Zheng, Xi, Lou, You-Rong R., Conney, Allan H., Maehr, Hubert, Adorini, Luciano, Uskokovic, Milan, and Suh, Nanjoo, "Gemini vitamin D ana-logues inhibit estrogen receptor-positive and estrogen recep-tor-negative mammary tumorigenesis without hypercalcemic toxicity," *Cancer Prevention Research (Philadelphia, Pa.)*, vol. 1, no. 6, 476–484 (2008).

29. Garland, Cedric F., Gorham, Edward D., Mohr, Sharif B., and Garland, Frank C., "Vitamin D for cancer prevention: global perspective," *Annals of Epidemiology*, vol. 19, no. 7, 468–483 (2009). Find the full article at http://www.annalsofepidemiology.org/article/PIIS1047279709001057/fulltext.

30. Cui, Yan, and Rohan, Thomas, "Vitamin D, calcium, and breast cancer risk: a review," *Cancer Epidemiology, Biomarkers, & Prevention*, vol. 15, no. 8, 1427 (2006). Find the full article at http://cebp.aacrjournals.org/content/15/8/1427.full.

31. See note 29.

32. Freedman, D. Michal, Looker, Anne C., Chang, Shih-Chen, and Graubard, Barry I., "Prospective study of serum vitamin D and cancer mortality in the United States," *Journal of the National Cancer Institute*, vol. 99, no. 21, 1594–1602 (2007). Get a PDF at http://www.direct-ms.org/pdf/VitDNonAuto/Freedman%20 Serum%20D%20Cancer%20UUS%20JNCI%202007.pdf.

33. See note 12.

34. McCullough, Marjorie, Stevens, Victoria, Patel, Roshni, Jacobs, Eric, Bain, Elizabeth, Horst, Ronald, Gapstur, Susan, Thun, Michael, and Calle, Eugenia, "Serum 25-hydroxyvitamin D concentrations and postmenopausal breast cancer risk: a nested case control study in the Cancer Prevention Study-II Nutrition Cohort," *Journal of Breast Cancer Research*, vol. 11, no. 4, 1465–5411 (2007). Get the full article at http://breast-cancer-research.com/content/11/4/R64.

35. Althuis, Michelle D., Fergenbaum, Jennifer H., Garcia-Closas, Montserrat, Brinton, Louise A., Madigan, M. Patricia, and Sherman, Mark E., "Etiology of hormone receptor-defined breast cancer: a systematic review of the literature," *Cancer Epidemiology, Biomarkers & Prevention*, vol. 13, no. 10, 1558–1568 (2004). Find a full copy at http://cebp.aacrjournals.org/content/13/10/1558.full.pdf.

36. Lew, Jasmine Q., Freedman, Neal D., Leitzmann, Michael F., Brinton, Louise A., Hoover, Robert N., Hollenbeck, Albert R., Schatzkin, Arthur, and Park, Yikyung, "Alcohol and risk of breast cancer by histologic type and hormone receptor status in postmenopausal women: the NIH-AARP Diet and Health Study," *American Journal of Epidemiology*, vol. 170, no. 3, 308–317 (2009).

37. Kabat, Geoffrey C., Kim, Mimi, Phipps, Amanda I., Li, Christopher I., Messina, Catherine R., Wactawski-Wende, Jean, Kuller, Lewis, Simon, Michael S., Yasmeen, Shagufta, Wassertheil-Smoller, Sylvia, and Rohan, Thomas E., "Smoking and alcohol consumption in relation to risk of triple-negative breast cancer in a cohort of postmenopausal women," *Cancer Causes and Control: CCC*, 1–9 (2011).

38. Li, Yan, Baer, David, Friedman, Gary D., Udaltsova, Natalia, Shim, Veronica, and Klatsky, Arthur L., "Wine, liquor, beer and risk of breast cancer in a large population," *European Journal of Cancer*, vol. 45, no. 5, 843–850 (2008).

39. Nielsen, Naja Rod, and Grønbæk, Morten, "Interactions between intakes of alcohol and postmenopausal hormones on risk of breast cancer," *International Journal of Cancer*, vol. 122, no. 5, 1109–1113 (2008).

40. Zhang, S. M., Willett, W. C., Selhub, J., Hunter, D. J., Giovannucci, E. L., Holmes, M. D., Colditz, G. A., and Hankinson, S. E. "Plasma folate, vitamin B6, vitamin B12, homocysteine, and risk of breast cancer," *Journal of the National Cancer Institute*, vol. 95, no. 14, 373–80 (2003). Find the full article at http://jnci.oxfordjournals.org/content/95/5/373.full.pdf.

41. Zhang, S., Hunter, D. J., Hankinson, S. E., Giovannucci, E. L., Rosner, B. A., Colditz, G. A., Speizer, F. E., and Willett, W. C., "A prospective study of folate intake and the risk of breast cancer," *JAMA: The Journal of the American Medical Association*, vol. 281, no. 17, 1632–1637 (1999). Find the full article at http://jama.ama-assn.org/content/281/17/1632.full.pdf.

42. Anders, Carey, "Understanding and treating triple-negative breast cancer," *Oncology*, vol. 22, no. 11, 1239–1240 (2008).

43. Bougnoux, P., Hajjaji, N., Ferrasson, M. N., Giraudeau, B., Couet, C., and Le Floch, O., "Improving outcome of chemotherapy of metastatic breast cancer by docosahexaenoic acid: a phase II trial," *British Journal of Cancer*, vol. 101, no. 12, 1978–1984 (2009). Find the full article at http://www.ncbi.nlm.nih.gov/pmc/articles/PMC2779856/.

44. Bonneterre, J., Dieras, V., Tubiana-Hulin, M., Bougnoux, P., Bonneterre, M. E., Delozier, T., Mayer, F., Culine, S., Dohoulou, N., and Bendahmane, B., "Phase II multicentre randomised study of docetaxel plus epirubicin *vs* 5-fluorouracil plus epirubicin and

cyclophosphamide in metastatic breast cancer," *British Journal of Cancer*, vol. 91, no. 8, 1466–1471 (2004). Find the full article at http://www.ncbi.nlm.nih.gov/pmc/articles/PMC2409942/.

45. Gago-Dominguez, M., Yuan, J.-M., Sun, C.-L., Lee, H.-P., and Yu, M. C., "Opposing effects of dietary n-3 and n-6 fatty acids on mammary carcinogenesis: the Singapore Chinese Health Study," *British Journal of Cancer*, vol. 89, no. 9, 1686–1692 (2003). Find the full article at http://www.nature.com/bjc/journal/v89/n9/full/6601340a.html.

46. Shu, Xiao Ou O., Zheng, Ying, Cai, Hui, Gu, Kai, Chen, Zhi, Zheng, Wei, and Lu, Wei, "Soy food intake and breast cancer survival," *JAMA: The Journal of the American Medical Association*, vol. 302, no. 22, 2437–2443 (2009). Find the full article at http://jama.ama-assn.org/content/302/22/2437.

47. "Human Health Issues," Environmental Protection Agency, http://www.epa.gov/pesticides/health/human.htm (accessed January 7, 2010).

48. "EWG's 2011 shopper's guide to pesticides in produce," Environmental Working Group, http://www.ewg.org/foodnews (accessed April 23, 2012).

49. The National Weight Control Registry is at http://www.nwcr.ws.

50. Chen, Qi, Espey, Michael G., Krishna, Murali C., Mitchell, James B., Corpe, Christopher P., Buettner, Garry R., Shacter, Emily, and Levine, Mark, "Pharmacologic ascorbic acid concentrations selectively kill cancer cells: action as a pro-drug to deliver hydrogen peroxide to tissues," *Proceedings of the National Academy of Sciences of the United States of America*, vol. 102, no. 38, 13604–13609 (2005). Find the full article at http://www.pnas.org/content/102/38/13604.full.

7

My Life Right Now

My hair comes back curly.

It begins to grow back a few weeks after I finish radiation, but at first it is just stubble. It does not become real hair for about four more months. Actual hair. Curly hair. I continue to wear a wig until I have about three-quarters of an inch of growth. Then I put the wigs in the closet, never to don them again. They're nice wigs and they tried hard, but I am so over them.

It is significant that this fact stands out in my mind: My hair comes back curly. I think this is because being bald was such a symbol of sickness to me. Having hair must mean I am well. Having curly hair must mean I am well plus mildly kinky.

Sadly, the hair straightens up within a year and I am kinky no more.

I ask my radiation oncologist, rather than a medical oncologist, to do my follow-up treatment. I choose her because I like the way she listens to my concerns and gives me thorough answers. And I like the office for reasons that really have little to do with her: Because radiation therapy is so tightly scheduled, with few emergencies to knock the timing off, I seldom run into other patients. The office is one level below the medical oncologists', so I am shielded from the memory of what I have just been through. The space is tranquil and welcoming, quiet and private.

And I settle into a new life full of doctors' visits. I see the radiation oncologist for a complete exam every six months. I get a mammogram and see my wonderful surgeon twice a year for the first three years, then yearly after that. I have blood work done with each visit. By staggering my visits, I see some doctor or another every three months. At first, this seems right, but eventually I tire of the constant stress of appointments.

My results are consistently normal, but I have become a hypochondriac, thinking every little symptom means I am sick again. It does not. I do not get sick again. I do not stop worrying about it, though.

When I return full time to school in the fall, the faculty and staff give me a bouquet of orchids. Dummy that I am, I have no idea what they are. *These are really pretty flowers,* I tell my assistant, Shari. Ever precise, Shari, who was the one who made the actual order, corrects me gently. *Well, actually, they are orchids.*

Oh, I say. *Wow, orchids,* I think. I begin to feel like Sally Field: *They like me, they really like me.*

At the first faculty meeting at which I preside, they clap for me. I am horribly embarrassed and terribly touched.

And then I get back to work. But I am not the same person. I have become a health food fanatic. No fried foods, no sugar, heavy on the vegetables, fruits, and complex carbs, minimal alcohol. People begin apologizing for their eating habits when I am around. If I catch a faculty or staff member eating potato chips or a candy bar, they make excuses.

I have become a food meanie, I think. People should feel free to eat what they eat, without answering to me. And then: *But really, potato chips?*

This healthier-than-thou attitude lasts a couple of years until I become less fearful, less constantly on my guard, less sure that one misstep and I will get cancer again. Bit by bit I let myself fall off the wagon occasionally. I have wine once or twice a week and a martini every Saturday night. I have French fries once a month or so. Do I know how to live, or what?

Still, eating well is what I can do to fight this disease, and I will do it. I have motivation I have never known before. And this ultimately makes me feel powerful rather than fearful—I am in control.

Right before diagnosis, I successfully dieted to lose weight, which was good. But I never counted my servings of vegetables and, if I did,

I would not have had to count very high. One.…After diagnosis, I am religious about five servings of fruits and vegetables. I once would eat broccoli only if it were smothered in cheese; now I eat it fresh, raw, and unadorned.

Joe continues to make me fresh vegetable juice every evening. Either he develops a better recipe or I get more accustomed to the drink—probably both—but I eventually start to actually like it. And I start each day with a green drink full of spirulina, alfalfa, wheat grass, mushrooms, green tea, and other healthy nutrients. It tastes like seaweed, so I gulp it down before I have a chance to wake up.

Initially, I take a boatload of vitamins—so many that my stomach eventually revolts and I reduce my intake to calcium, B-complex, vitamin D, omega-3, and CoQ10. I figure I eat well enough to not need a multivitamin. I later add glucosamine-chondroitin for my aching bones; it helps, and I read initial research that says chondroitin may be a cancer-fighter, especially against metastatic triple negative. Yay.

My diet is mostly vegetarian with some fish. I allow myself meat occasionally, but find that I seldom miss it. And the more I go without it, the more difficult it is for me to digest it. There is a message there from my stomach, I think. It is happier without meat.

I return to the personal trainer I had hired before my diagnosis and finish the session I had already paid for before I got sick. But I am weakened and my muscles ache. I eventually quit—I have, after all, more than surpassed my original goal. I had told him I wanted to lose 20 pounds and, over two years, I dropped 50. I can now wear clothes from before I was married in 1970. Conveniently, they are again in fashion.

I continue exercising—walking when we are in Iowa, and hiking in Colorado. And I keep the weight off. I have learned a great deal about training—that I have to push myself for it to have effect, and that what I had once considered exercise was only slightly better than sitting on a couch. I strive for at least four hours a week of exercise that makes me sweat.

Even with my emphasis on health through physical activity and nutrition, though, I remain frustratingly tired. If it is true that you generally should expect a recovery time at least as long as your treatment time, I should feel better in four months. I don't. I do gradually gain more energy, but I am far from energetic.

Is this because I am in my 60s—I was 60 at diagnosis—and I would have felt like this without cancer? Who knows? I don't dwell on it; instead, I keep active and keep my mind and body focused on other things.

My surgical incision hurts occasionally, a sharp pain that points to where the tumor was. The doctor says this is because of nerve damage from surgery. Early on I sometimes get shooting pains in my chest wall, but these go away. Nobody knows for sure what they are all about—perhaps a reaction to the radiation.

I do gentle arm exercises every night to reduce the threat of lymphedema—swinging one arm in a circle, and then the next, first forward, then backward; reaching into space with the left hand then with the right. The surgical incision in my armpit occasionally hurts, but gradually the pain disappears.

I find that I occasionally have slight memory problems, such as trouble thinking of a word. But my life as a teacher and writer helps me with synonyms. If I can't think of *Adirondack chair*, I can remember the less precise *deck chair*. I tell my brother Ed I think I have chemobrain. "Oh, you just have Prijatel brain," he jokes, insisting that he has the same problem.

Bless him. There's that normalcy again.

My memory does get better. I write an article on the subject and learn that some researchers believe memory loss may be the result of changes in the brain caused by cancer itself, rather than by its treatment. If my memory has improved, maybe that means the cancer is truly and finally gone.

Eventually the stress of the job returns. I often spend the night worrying rather than sleeping, so I start the day already tired. That, added to being drained from treatment, means I have many days when I am just plain exhausted. Long ago, I got a cozy easy chair for my office, so I shut my door and take a power nap occasionally. It gets me through the day.

I am now an administrator, and the teaching portion of my job—the part that I love—has been pushed to a corner. I teach one class, so most of my interaction with students is on committees and with complaints.

I grow restless. I feel it is time to do something else. I have learned so much about this disease and health in general that I believe I should focus on sharing that knowledge.

So I decide to retire at the end of the year, in May, a year after diagnosis, and return to my first love: writing. I have always thought being a health writer would be a satisfying life, so that is where I head.

I miss the students. I will always miss the students. Any teacher worth her salt will always miss the students. Still, I know I do not have the energy I once had to teach with the passion I expect of myself. I refuse to be one of those teachers who *used* to be good. If I can't maintain my high standards, I will stay out of the classroom.

And I begin writing this book, a task that will take roughly forever and three weeks.

I begin my blog, *Positives About Negative,* to counter the dismal projections I read about this disease. Perhaps I can help others. At any rate, I seriously educate myself.

Within two years, my radiation oncologist takes another job out of state and I ask my primary care physician to do my follow-up. I love this choice. She is exceptional, so I feel she will find what needs to be found. And she looks at my entire body, not just my breast. That makes me feel like a full person, not just a diseased boob.

Seeing a Regular Person's Doctor makes me view myself as a regular person, surrounded by people getting flu shots and talking about bursitis. I do not feel the hint of death around me. I feel health. I feel like me. Plain me, not cancer me.

I create a bucket list long enough to take many years to finish. Bit by bit, I tick items off:

Go to Alaska. Check. We do that right after I retire, taking ferries up the Inside Passage and wandering around islands and inlets, watching black bears and grizzlies, enjoying the crystalline ocean, frontier cities, and staggering mountain vistas. We fly to Anchorage and drive up to Mt. McKinley. It is beautiful, restful, invigorating.

Go to Yellowstone. Check. We do that the next year, staying in a hotel right by Old Faithful. I call my kids, both now in their 30s, and apologize for never taking them there. It is a scientific marvel, with hot springs and geysers amidst craggy mountain peaks and heart-stopping waterfalls.

Spend more time with the people who are important to me—my family and friends. Check. I make a conscious effort to reach out to people touched by cancer, which is way too many people I know. I lose good friends to cancers of all types, and I am happy that I spent time with them beforehand and offered comfort.

Climb the mountain by our cabin. Check. Well, I make it to tree line, the point at which the trail turns to boulders, about 10,500 feet, which was my intention. Joe, Josh, and I go together, and Josh makes it all the way to the top—12,600 feet—by the time Joe and I make it to tree line. Afterward, we eat massive amounts of Mexican food at a nearby restaurant to celebrate.

Go to Machu Picchu. Check. I saved this one for my fifth-year anniversary after diagnosis. Joe and I go with my nephew Russ on a 10-day excursion for which I have extremely high expectations. The trip exceeds them. It is literally breathtaking—we are at heights from 8,000 to 14,000 feet, so I spend a good deal of the time gasping for breath. But the country is one marvel after another—the Andes, Inca ruins on granite cliffs, an azure mountain lake at 12,000 feet with natives living on islands they built from reeds, famers in native garb harvesting fields by hand.

I have plenty of items left on the list—the Dalmatian Coast, Cinque Terre, a compost pile, painting more. But I have time.

I have time. Hear that? I have time.

Three years after my diagnosis, I finally start to get angry that I had cancer. One catalyst for this anger is that I come across the statistics from the National Cancer Institute estimating that 12.7 percent of all women will face breast cancer in their lives. So that means that 87.3 percent of all women will *not* face breast cancer.

After being positive and upbeat and shrugging this thing off for years, I start to ask, "Why me?"

But why after so long?

I think I used all my positive energy to fight this thing and, years later, only begin feeling safe enough to get cranky about being selected for this elite club.

This anger also comes at a time when I am facing my various doctors' visits and mammograms and blood tests and whatever else might crop up.

I am tired of it. Tired of these regular worries about what might come. *Are they going to find something this year? Has it come back after all this time?*

Remaining positive is wearing on me. Joe says there is no reason to think they will find anything at this point—I am feeling fine and have no symptoms. But, I tell him, if there is no risk, why do they do the tests at all?

I remember so many friends who passed their tests and then ended up with a cough, a bump, a whatever, and the nasty stuff was back.

Yet, others catch something early and take care of it.

Because my original diagnosis was not as frightening as most, I sometimes feel that I am not as justified in complaining as others. A friend tells me that somebody had called hers a "fake cancer" because it was hormone-positive and less than a centimeter. But, even though she has a better prognosis, she still faces the possibility of cancer returning. We all do. It happened once, and we are forever on our guard.

That stinks.

Plus, I wonder, if this did come back, what would I do? Go through chemo again? I am truly not sure. I might just take my savings and hop a plane to travel the world. Or a boat. Probably a boat.

I honestly do worry less and less about getting sick. Weeks go by without my obsessing that something is amiss with my body.

A few weeks after the fourth anniversary of my diagnosis, I break my elbow—actually, I fracture my radius, one of the elbow bones. It's the result of a fairly spectacular fall during an otherwise lovely walk. I step on the sidewalk wrong and fall first on one shoulder, then another, then one knee and another, then the elbow.

I must look like an empty beer can being tossed around the beach in the wind. Thump. Splat. Bang. Bump.

Both shoulders are bruised and both knees horribly scraped. I have water with me, so I wash myself off and put a Kleenex on the knees to stop the bleeding. I figure that is my biggest problem, as my elbow barely hurts.

Stunningly, a couple across the street is out working in their front yard and they do not offer help—they do not even acknowledge me, sitting on the sidewalk tending to my wounds. Finally, I feel OK, and Joe helps me stand up. We walk home, a little more slowly than before. I shoot the couple a look. They stare down at their rakes.

At home, I shower and clean myself up, bandage the knees, and wrap the elbow, which is beginning to hurt. By the next morning, I cannot straighten my arm, so we head to the emergency room—it is Memorial Day, and no doctors' offices are open.

I think of Elizabeth Edwards, moving furniture and breaking a rib, which led to the discovery that her cancer had metastasized. Did my elbow break easily because of cancer? Hardly, I tell my hypochondriac self. I fell on almost every part of my body the sidewalk could reach, and all I did was hurt my elbow. Actually, that probably means my bones are pretty strong.

Turns out the bones are fine. It is just a hairline fracture and it does not require a cast—a wrap and a sling are enough. The elbow hurts a bit—certainly not what you would expect with a fractured elbow—but it is not much of a problem. Yoga is difficult—no downward facing dogs for me. Ouch. And typing is a little painful, so I have to slow my writing down a bit. I should be fine in a month, the doc says. And I am—the elbow heals nicely, and I hit the yoga mat and put on the dog with no problems.

I am almost glad I did it, as it provided proof to me that my bones are healthy.

But the drama is not over. Within a week of the fall, we head to the Colorado cabin, where we have a great few weeks until one evening when I get extremely lightheaded, weak on one side, have trouble breathing, and feel like I am about to pass out. I drink water to hydrate myself, thinking it is dehydration, and snack on fruit, thinking it might be a blood sugar issue. It doesn't help.

When I hurt my arm, I remember the nurse at the emergency room saying there had been some internal bleeding by the fracture. Do I now have a blood clot moving toward my brain? Or, of course, the inevitable worry: Has the cancer moved to the brain? That's a fairly common destination for triple-negative.

Joe drives me to the hospital in Walsenburg, nearly an hour trip from our cabin, but still the closest clinic. I try to relax, breathe deeply, inhale air through the open car window. But I continue to feel like I will soon pass out. My left side is only slightly numb, but numb nevertheless. And it is the left elbow I fractured.

We arrive at about 7 p.m. I do not practice what I will say to the doctor, which is a mistake, as when I walk in to the emergency room, all I can say is I feel "weird" and my left side is weak. The doctor asks for specifics, and I repeat the ever-so-helpful and precise "weird."

He asks my occupation, and when I tell him I am a retired journalism professor and a health writer, he seems to think I should speak clearer than that.

He asks me to say "Mississippi," and I work hard to articulate, as though I am drunk. He then asks me to say "Four forty four fours." I tell him I never have been able to pronounce "r"s well, and that my brother used to tease me when I said "poach."

"But there are no 'r's in poach," he says.

Later, I realize I should have clarified that my brother teased me because I had been trying to say "porch."

They hook me up to an IV and monitor my vitals. My blood pressure, which normally is low (110/65), spikes (145/109).

I have enough possible symptoms of a stroke, or a TIA—transient ischemic attack—to cause the doctor to worry. A CAT scan shows my brain is OK, but he is concerned that the machine is not precise enough, and if I am at risk of a stroke, he wants to prevent it.

"Early intervention is critical," he says. "We want you to keep returning to your cabin for another 20 years." After 20 years, apparently they want me out.

He calls a stroke specialist in Denver, and they agree that I need to go to the stroke center there.

"We'll helicopter you," he says.

"Yikes," I say.

The copter comes from Pueblo with two excellent paramedics, who strap me onto a board and load me right next to the pilot. My feet are touching the front of the glass bubble. To my left is nothing but glass and sky; the pilot is to my right. I can see his GPS system showing us where we are and where we are headed.

Or, rather, I could have seen it if I had my glasses. I am blurry-eyed, though, because I can take nothing on board with me—not my purse, shoes, watch. The only possession I keep is my underwear—and it, of course, is old and slightly tattered. I had been at a cabin in the wilderness and felt no need for fancy pants. Too bad. I am a stereotype—in the hospital with crummy undies.

As I fly north, over Pueblo and Colorado Springs on a clear June night, my main worry is that the cancer has returned in my brain. Oddly, I am ready to accept the inevitable. That is probably the Valium they had given me, though, to calm me for the ride. *If I die,* I think, *I die.*

Such drama.

In Denver, I have a second scan, this one including the arteries in my neck. Then I have a brain MRI and an echocardiogram. All are normal.

At 2 a.m., I finally see a doctor, who tells me he does not think I've had a stroke, but that they want to keep me for observation because they don't know what the problem is. I am transferred from the ER to a hospital room, where I fall happily asleep for an hour and a half—until a nurse comes to draw my blood.

Meanwhile, Joe has driven up to Denver, stopping in Pueblo to pick up my sister Phyllis, who I knew would keep him awake during the trip. They arrive pie-eyed from lack of sleep. Joe has had no dinner. He finally eats later in the morning, 16 hours after his last meal. Phyllis brings me a change of clothes, but Joe has the same work clothes he wore when he drove me to the hospital.

The neurologist finally visits in early afternoon, and we talk about my medical history. I mention the breast cancer, and he orders a second MRI with a more precise reading, to see if the cancer had spread.

It hasn't.

I say, "Yay!" But I still have no idea what my problem is. Nor, apparently, do the doctors. The only out-of-whack reading in all my tests is a slightly low potassium level and the high blood pressure.

By 4 p.m., my blood pressure is back down to normal and the docs see no more need for me to be hospitalized. The concluding diagnosis: a complex migraine. That sounds to me like a fallback position—better than saying, "We have no idea." I do some research on complex migraines and remain unconvinced. I had only a slight headache—not migraine-level.

So, I am released and we head back to our mountain cabin, subdued, concerned, and confused.

For several weeks afterward, I am leery of my health. As Joe and I hike, I am haunted by the possibility that my head or my heart or my something will go out and—whap—I will die facedown in a cow pie. I feel fine, though, and we intensify our hikes, and I continue to feel fine.

What happened? I will continue to ask that question, and, eventually, I might find an answer. Some speculations: The trapped blood in my elbow fracture had come loose and moved toward my brain, but broke up before it did damage. The docs, though, seemed unconcerned about any connection between my symptoms and my arm.

Or another: We had been in town that day and I'd had more than my usual caffeine. I had three diet Cokes with lunch. Plus, I think the decaf coffee I ordered actually had caffeine—two shots. And the temperature was in the mid-90s. Could I have had dehydration plus excess caffeine? Low potassium is one sign of dehydration.

Because my symptoms were classic ones for stroke, I think the docs looked for the obvious and did not evaluate the more esoteric issues. That appears to be another medical mystery for me to solve.

One thing I do now know, though, is that my cancer has not spread to my brain. But I also realize cancer is not the only thing that can kill me. I have spent so much time in the past few years focused on dying of cancer than I now see that I have to broaden my horizons. Hey, I could die of just about anything.

Good to know.

This realization is oddly freeing. It helps me become less cancer-phobic. I have complained that doctors during treatment saw me as only a breast. Well, I now see that I have not been much better. I have seen me through the lens of cancer.

That cancer is gone, and it has been gone for years. Time to move on. Something is going to kill me eventually, but looking over my shoulder and waiting for it defines my life by fear. Cancer changed me in ways I still probably don't understand. But it did not kill my body. And I will not let it kill my spirit.

What Cancer Means to Me Now

I sometimes play the "what if" game. What if I had never moved to Iowa? What if I had had more kids? What if I had been born rich? What if I had never had cancer?

There has never been much future in that game, and adding the cancer card makes it no more fulfilling or fun. I have no idea how my life would have been different without cancer. I do know I am a different person than I was before I got sick, and I like this person better. She has a much broader view of what life means than she did before she was sick.

I am more introspective, more understanding, more thoughtful. I was OK in these areas before, but I feel cancer added another layer to my personality, an ability to look deeper, to care more about others, to see what I had been blind to before—that my life is good and it is up to me to keep it that way and, perhaps, try to make it better.

I will never consider cancer a gift, although others say they see it that way. I do have to acknowledge that it has made me live a more rewarding life. I wish I could have done that on my own, without this scare, but I didn't.

Cancer was not a blessing, but it did help me see the blessings that surround me—my family and friends, my career, my mind, my overall health.

I eat healthier, I exercise more purposefully, I do yoga, I meditate. Joe and I find a new church and, through it, become a part of a community that makes me think about small moments and big responsibilities and how I live my life as a good person. I drink less. I see my acupuncturist regularly, just because she calms me so much.

And that's the word. Calm. I feel so much calmer than I ever have in my life. I get there through meditation and prayer and talking with good friends and family and by taking deep breaths. I get there by looking at the beauty around me and just enjoying it. Not trying to redo it as I used to, not trying to judge it. Just enjoying it. Just being.

Three years after diagnosis, my first grandchild, Tarin Gram, is born. Eighteen months later, we welcome his brother Eli Finn.

I am so grateful that I have seen the birth of these two beautiful little boys who are, of course, smart in addition to being cuter than anybody else's grandbabies. And I plan to be around to see them grow up.

I happily return to the classroom part time, and do several writing workshops, so I am once again in the midst of students.

So all is good.

But I really wish my hair had stayed curly.

TNBC Women

The women I have met throughout this book, I believe, are the best elixir against my worries. We have all survived, and we are, perhaps, a bit more appreciative of our lives because we were faced with the reality of our own deaths. This life is no longer to be taken for granted. It is to be cherished, enjoyed, lived well.

I see Rebecca a few times a year. She is a "neighbor" at our Colorado cabin—it's about a 40-minute drive to get from her place to ours, but a crow could probably take a few minutes to wing the roughly four miles of meadow and foothills. Rebecca comes up to ride horses with my sister-in-law Gwyn, and we sometimes talk. Rebecca looks good;

she looks content. She talks about the baby she was nursing when she was diagnosed; she has seen him past his 30th birthday.

Pat Jones is perhaps the story that quells my worries the most—she and her daughter Candy have shared three bouts with hormone-negative. And Pat shows that a second cancer can be beaten, just like the first. I still see Pat's messages occasionally in chat rooms, where she encourages other women with her story. Nearly 25 years past her first diagnosis and nine years past her second, she demonstrates resiliency and is proof that this disease is not an automatic killer. Candy is also celebrating more than ten years cancer-free.

I regularly send these women e-mails asking for updates. The responses have been delightful. Rosa sent me a wedding photo. Melody talked about her pregnancy, the fulfillment of a desire she had wistfully expressed in our first interview. Julie told me about finishing more triathlons.

I become Facebook friends with Lynda, who posts remarkable photos of the Colorado plains at sunrise, in snowstorms, with storm clouds gathering, and wildfires burning in the distance. I hope to meet her on one of our drives to Colorado, as her ranch is on the way. Noreen often sends me research updates, especially on environmental influences on cancer.

These are the faces of triple-negative—young mothers and grandmothers, black and white and brown, from the East, West, North, South, and Midwest. Worriers and warriors. Plain women living meaningful lives long after cancer intersected their paths, some changed remarkably, some only marginally, some in barely discernable ways.

We're not heroes; we're not victims. We are just women who, like all other women in the world, are trying to put one foot in front of the other and get through the day. Dealing with the present, looking forward to the future.

Appendix
Annotated Pathology Report: Pat's Case

I HAD TWO SURGICAL PATHOLOGY REPORTS—ONE FROM the initial biopsy that diagnosed my cancer and a second from the complete excision of the tumor by partial mastectomy, or lumpectomy. The original, or initial diagnostic surgical pathology, report was much shorter than the more comprehensive "definitive treatment" surgical pathology report. Most surgeons and oncologists rely on the report generated from the definitive (final) surgical specimen because there is a greater volume of tumor on which to base the pathological assessment. An interpretation of the two reports:

Diagnostic Report: Specimen

A. Breast biopsy left 12:00

B. Breast biopsy 3:00

The numbers refer to a clock-like placement of the trouble spots the radiologist noticed on an ultrasound. One was right above my nipple, at the high noon position. The other was at mid-afternoon, or 3 o'clock.

Diagnostic Report: Gross Description

> A: Labeled—left breast cores 12:00 is a 1.5 × 0.6 × 0.2 cm aggregate of tan-pink tissue cores and core fragments.
>
> B: Labeled—left breast cores 3:00 is a 1 × 0.4 × 0.2 cm aggregate of pink-yellow tissue cores including blood clots.

The tumor was 1.5 cm at its largest, so the pathologist called it a 1.5-cm tumor, making it early stage. I had two tissue samples taken. The second, which was not cancerous, was 1 cm at the largest.

Diagnostic Report: Diagnosis

> A: Breast, left at 12:00, biopsy: poorly differentiated infiltrating ductal carcinoma (Bloom-Richardson high grade) with possible capillary lymphatic space involvement.
>
> B: Breast, left at 3:00, biopsy: blood clot and benign stromal fragments.

This was a bad news–good news section. The bad was that I had cancer. It was *ductal* and had broken through the duct wall, so it was spreading, or *infiltrating*. And it was high grade, or aggressive. However, the second suspicious site the doctor found was benign. It was a simple blood clot with fragments of the connective tissue of the breast, or *stroma*.

Surgical Report: Specimen

> A. Sentinel lymph node biopsy
>
> B. Breast biopsy eval surgical margins
>
> C. Lymph node regional resection

The *sentinel node* is the lymph node to which the cancer is most likely to spread. Doctors identify it by putting dye into your breast before surgery, close to the tumor. The dye will head to the sentinel node and help the surgeon easily find it. *Surgical margins* refers to the cancer-free zone between the tumor and the edge of the excision. *Lymph node regional resection* describes the procedure used to remove the lymph nodes for study.

Surgical Report: Clinical History

> *Left breast cancer.*

The original biopsy had diagnosed cancer, so the pathologist went in knowing what he was dealing with.

Surgical Report: Dr. Consultation

> *Dr. Docktor: B: left breast—1.3 cm tumor 0.3 cm from deep margin.*

The pathologist's name (changed for legal purposes), plus his measurement of my tumor. It measured smaller (1.3 cm) after surgery than on my mammogram (1.5 cm).

Surgical Report: Frozen Section Diagnosis

> *Dr. Docktor: AF1, AF2–AF39(m)—left axillary sentinel node #1—there is no evidence of malignancy.*

The pathologist's name (changed again) and statement on my sentinel lymph nodes status. The cancer had not spread! Yay, good news!

Surgical Report: Gross Description

> *A: Labeled "left axillary sentinel node #1" are three, 2.2 × 1.2 × 1.3 cm (#1), 1.8 × 1.2 × 1 cm (#2), and 1.5 × 1.1 × 0.8 cm (#3) lymph nodes, each discolored with blue dye.*

AF1: Lymph node #1

AF2: Lymph node #2

AF3: Lymph node #3

B: Labeled "left breast tissue" is a 6.6 × 6.8 × 2.2 cm portion of breast tissue with a localization needle in place. There are multifocal calcifications and a stereotactic clip adjacent to the localization needle and identified on the accompanying mammogram. The margins are inked. Sections reveal a 1.3 × 1.1 × 1.2 cm gray stellate mass lesion that focally extends to within 0.3 cm of the nearest (deep) margin and is adjacent to a biopsy cavity. The biopsy cavity contains white pellet-like material. Focal fibrous breast parenchyma is found away from the biopsy cavity and the residual mass.

B1–B2: Mass lesion and deep margin.

B3: Central aspect of mass lesion.

B4: Fibrous parenchyma adjacent to mass lesion.

C: Labeled "additional axillary tissue left" is a 6.2 × 4.3 × 1.3 cm. aggregate of fat. Sections reveal possible lymph nodes ranging from 0.3 to 0.7 cm in maximum dimension (entire whole lymph nodes, 3).

I had three lymph nodes removed; this section gives their total dimensions. It also describes how much of my breast was removed. The *localization needle* refers to the needle that was placed in my breast during a mammogram before surgery, to pinpoint the exact location of my tumor. This is extremely helpful when there is a large amount of breast tissue and the tumor is tiny. The tumor's greatest dimension was 1.3 cm. The other data describe my tissue.

Surgical Report: Microscopic Description

The sentinel lymph node shows no evidence of metastatic carcinoma.

The left breast tissue shows residual comedocarcinoma both in situ and invasive. [Comedocarcinoma is a term that is generally reserved for in situ cancers, so this might have been included because of concerns that, in addition to the tumor, I might have also had DCIS.] The tumor does not approach the inked surgical margin. I see no evidence of vascular or lymphatic invasion. The surrounding breast parenchyma shows adenosis without dysplasia or tumor.

The C tissue is predominantly fatty with a small lymph node. No metastatic carcinoma is encountered.

Estrogen receptor assays were performed on prior material. The tumor was estrogen receptor negative, weakly positive for progesterone receptor assay and negative for Her-2/neu. The maximum size of the tumor on mammogram was 2.1 cm.

Comedocarcinoma refers to the pattern of ductal breast cancer. The rest of my milk ducts—the *parenchyma*—are free of cancer. Adenosis is a benign growth; *without dysplasia* means there are no premalignant abnormalities. My tumor was ER-negative; weakly PR-positive, and Her2-negative. These tests had not been done on my original biopsy. The reference to the mammogram has always confused me, as the mammogram showed a 1.5-cm tumor.

Surgical Report: Diagnosis

A: Left axillary sentinel node: Negative for metastatic carcinoma.

B. Left breast cancer showing:

1. Evidence of prior surgery.

2. Residual infiltrating and intraductal comedocarcinoma.

3. No evidence of vascular or lymphatic invasion.

4. Maximum tumor size on mammogram 2.1.

5. No evidence of vascular or lymphatic invasion.

6. Adequate surgical margins.

An overview of prior information.

Surgical Report: Microscopic

Size of Invasive Component

Greatest dimension: 1.1 cm.

Comment: If there is a discrepancy between gross and microscopic tumor measurement, the microscopic measurement of the invasive component takes precedence and should be use fro tumor staging.

The gross description had defined my tumor as 1.3 at the largest; here it says 1.1, and says that this number should be the one used for treatment planning. I'm all for the smaller number. That's the one my oncologist circled.

Histologic Type

Invasive ductal carcinoma with an extensive intraductal component.

The cancer type, and a statement that it had broken through the duct wall.

Histologic Grade

NOTTINGHAM HISTOLOGIC SCORE

Mitotic count:

For a 40× objective with a field area of 0.152 mm2

0 to 5 mitoses per 10 HPF (score = 1)

6 to 10 mitoses per 10 HPF (score = 2)

Greater than 10 mitoses per 10 HPF (score = 3)

Total Nottingham Score:

Grade II: 6–7 points

These findings indicated a favorable revision of my tumor grade, and therefore my prognosis. My original biopsy, which used the Bloom-Richardson scale, demonstrated an aggressive tumor. The definitive surgical specimen, however, which was tested using the Nottingham Histologic Score, was more consistent with a cancer of an intermediate aggressive potential.

Surgical Report: Extent of Invasion

Primary Tumor (pT)

pT1: Tumor 2.0 cm or less in greatest dimension

Regional Lymph Nodes (pN)

pN0: No regional lymph node metastasis histologically (ie, none greater than 0.2 mm). No additional examination for isolated tumor cells.

Specify: Number examined: 1

Number involved: 0

Distant Metastasis (M)

pMX: Cannot be assessed

Margins

Margins uninvolved by invasive carcinoma. Distance from closest margin: 0.3 cm.

For staging purposes, my cancer was pT1, pN0, pMX. Early stage, with no involved lymph nodes, and no signs of metastases but no guarantee that the cancer had not spread elsewhere. The margins were clear, meaning surgery had successfully removed all of the cancerous tumor.

All in all, for hormone-negative diagnosis, this was not bad. I had a small—1.1 cm—invasive ductal carcinoma, or a cancerous tumor that had broken through the duct wall. It had not spread to the lymph nodes, and there was no sign of other metastases, although small cells could have broken away and not been seen. The two tests of tumor aggression were mixed. The original biopsy had diagnosed a high-grade tumor according to the Bloom-Richardson scale. The surgical report, though, used the Nottingham Histologic Score; my tumor was of medium aggression there. The tumor was estrogen-receptor-negative, weakly positive for progesterone, and Her2/neu-negative. According to some doctors, the weakly positive progesterone reading kept me out of the triple-negative, or highly aggressive, category. To others, weakly positive means negative, so they consider me triple-negative. Nowhere in my reports, however, is the term *triple-negative* used, although my diagnosis came at a time when TNBC was newly named. My surgical margins were clear by 0.3 cm, a tumor-free zone large enough to constitute negative margins. My wonderful surgeon had successfully removed all of the cancer from my breast.

Glossary

AC: Chemotherapy using Adriamycin, an anthracycline, and Cytoxan, an alkalating agent.

Accelerated partial breast radiation: A shortened course of high-dose radiation focused only on the lumpectomy site.

ACT: Chemotherapy using an anthracycline and an alkylating agent, plus a taxane—usually Andriamycin and Cytoxan first, followed by paclitaxel or docetaxel.

Adjuvant chemotherapy: Chemotherapy given after surgery.

ALDH1: A genetic marker for breast cancer tissue that is associated with an especially serious prognosis.

Alkylating drugs, or platinum agents: Drugs that attack the DNA of cancer cells, creating a platinum complex inside the cancer cell that ultimately kills it. This includes cyclophosphamide (Cytoxan), carboplatin (Paraplatin) and cisplatin (Platinol-AQ and Platinu).

Androgens: Normally considered male hormones, the most common being testosterone, that are also present in women's bodies.

Aneuploid tumors: A type of tumor that is associated with chromosome abnormalities and may indicate a form of breast cancer that is inheritable.

Anthracylines, or antitumor antibiotics: Drugs that prevent cancer cell division by disrupting the structure of the DNA. They include doxorubicin (Adriamycin) and epirubicin (Ellence).

Antimetabolites: Drugs that kill cancer by interfering with the metabolic process. These include fluorouracil, or 5-FU or f5U (Adrucil, Carac, Efudex, and Fluoroplex) and capecitabine (Xeloda).

Arimidex: An aromatase inhibitor, a drug that lowers the level of estrogen in the body. It is often given to postmenopausal women with hormone-positive disease. It is not used for hormone-negative breast cancer or TNBC.

Aurora-A: An enzyme important to healthy cell proliferation.

Axillary lymph nodes: Lymph nodes in the armpits.

Axillary lymph node dissection: Removal of all cancerous armpit nodes.

Basal-like breast cancers: Cancers that grows in the basal layer of the breast, the outer layer that lines the mammary ducts. Associated with triple-negative breast cancer.

Bisphenol A (BPA): Chemical found in the lining of metal food cans and plastic containers that has been connected to many types of cancer in animals.

Bloom-Richardson scale: A measure of tumor aggressiveness. Low-grade means the cells look almost normal and are less aggressive; high-grade means the cells look less like normal cells and are probably more aggressive and fast-growing.

BMI, or body mass index: A measurement of the amount of fat in your body. In general, if your number is below 21, you are underweight; between 21 and 24.9, you are normal; between 25 and 29.9 and you are overweight; above 30, you are obese.

Breast magnetic resonance imaging (MRI): The use of magnetic signals to provide information on the internal makeup of breast tissue.

BRCA: Breast cancer gene. Can be either BRCA1 or BRCA2. Mutations of the gene are associated with breast cancer, especially triple-negative breast cancer.

Bilateral mastectomy: Removal of both breasts. Also called a *double mastectomy*.

Biopsy: Removal of a small sample of breast tissue that can be tested for cancer.

Brachytherapy: Radiation treatment using radiated beads implanted in the tumor site and left for five days.

Calcifications: Calcium deposits in the breasts. Larger deposits, called *macrocalcifications,* are typically benign. Clusters of tiny deposits, called *microcalcifications,* can be suspicious and may require a biopsy.

Chemopause: Chemotherapy shuts down the ovaries in premenopausal women causing chemically induced menopause.

Claudin-low breast cancer: A newly defined molecular subtype of breast cancer that is usually triple-negative and shows a tendency to metastasize.

Clear margins: The most successful lumpectomies are those with clear, or negative, margins. This means that the cancer has not extended beyond the edge of the tissue taken.

Close margins: A minimal amount of cancerous tissue at the edges of a specimen taken during surgery.

CMF: Chemotherapy that combines Cytoxan, methotrexate (Amethopterin, Mexate, Folex), and fluorouracil (5FU).

Complete pathological response: Applies to surgery after neoadjuvant therapy; all clinical evidence of the tumor is gone—there is no sign of the cancer after surgery.

Contralateral mastectomy: Removal of the opposite, or unaffected, breast.

Core needle biopsy: Use of a needle to remove tissue samples from a lump.

Cytokeratin 5/6: Proteins in the body's epithelial cells, or cells lining our internal organs, membranes, skin, and glands, that are highly correlated with basal-like breast cancers.

DEAR1 gene: A gene that develops in the ducts of the breast and in the glands and may be connected to TNBC.

Disease-free survival: Survival after a specific time with no sign of disease; also called *relapse-free survival.*

Distant metastasis: Any spread of breast cancer to a site outside the breast.

Dose-dense chemotherapy (DDC): Chemotherapy every two weeks.

Ductal breast cancer: Cancer that originates in the ducts that carry the milk through the breast to the nipple. Also called *ductal carcinoma.*

Ductal carcinoma in situ: Ductal breast cancer that has not spread, but remains within the milk duct; usually considered precancer.

Epidermal growth factor receptor (EGFR): Also called Her1, EGFR belongs to a family of receptors that includes Her2, Her3, and Her4. It binds to cells and is part of a system that regulates cell growth and development and is associated with basal-like breast cancer.

EGFR inhibitors: Drugs that interfere with the epidermal growth factor receptor. These include erlotinib, cetuximab, and panitumumab (Tarceva, Erbitux, and Vectibix).

Estrogen: A hormone produced primarily by the ovaries and, during pregnancy, the placenta; other sources of small amounts are the adrenal glands, liver, and breasts. In postmenopausal women, estrogen is produced by fat cells.

Estrogen-receptor-negative breast cancer: Lacking receptors for the hormone estrogen.

External beam radiation: X-rays directly aimed at the site of the breast tumor and nearby tissue. It is usually given five days a week for six weeks.

EZH2 stem cells: The protein EZH2 is expressed in a great majority of hormone-receptor-negative tumors, mostly triple-negative.

Fine needle aspiration: A type of biopsy in which the doctor uses a small needle, similar to that used for a blood sample, to extract cells or liquid from a lump.

Fluorescence in situ hybridization (FISH): A genetic test that compares the number of Her2 genes to normal genes. More than two Her2 genes for each normal gene indicates a cancer that is Her2-positive.

Her2/neu: Human epidermal growth factor receptor 2.

Her2-positive: Cancers that are positive for the epidermal growth factor receptor 2, or Her2/neu.

Herceptin: A drug commonly used for Her2-positive breast cancers.

High-dose chemotherapy (HDCT): An aggressive regimen that can destroy bone marrow along with cancer cells.

Histopathology: The microscopic study of abnormal tissue as a result of disease.

Histologic grade: How abnormal the cells look to a pathologist, which is a measure of tumor aggressiveness.

Histologic type: The cell type of a tumor—*ductal* or *lobular*. This also describes the growth pattern: If the cells fill the duct, the pattern is *solid*; if the cells grow in fingers, the pattern is *papillary*.

Hormone-negative breast cancer: General term for breast cancers that are negative for estrogen and progesterone receptors.

Hormone receptors: Proteins in cells that bind to hormones. Breast cells with receptors bind and react to either estrogen or progesterone, or both.

Immunohistochemistry (IHC): A test of antigens (proteins) in tissue, which can help diagnose cancer by identifying microorganisms related to cancer.

Inflammatory breast cancer: Cancer that usually does not form as a tumor, but rather as a swelling or thickening of the breast.

Insulin-like growth factor receptor 1 (IGF-1R): A receptor that mediates the effects of the protein hormone IGF-1, which is similar in structure to insulin and may be overexpressed in many cases of triple-negative breast cancer.

Insulin resistance: A condition in which the body produces insulin but does not use it properly.

Invasive ductal cancer: Cancer that has broken through the duct wall and begun to spread. Also called *invasive ductal carcinoma*.

Invasive lobular cancer: Cancer that has spread outside the lobules. Also called *invasive lobular carcinoma*.

Lobular breast cancer: Cancer that develops in the lobules, where milk is formed. Also called *lobular carcinoma*.

Luminal A: Breast cancer that is ER-positive, PR-positive, and Her2-negative.

Luminal B: Breast cancer that is ER-positive, PR-positive, and Her2-positive.

Lumpectomy: Also called a *partial mastectomy*, a lumpectomy takes only the cancerous portion of the breast, plus enough surrounding tissue to ensure removal of the entire tumor. Other terms for this operation include *breast conservation surgery, quadrantectomy, segmental excision, wide excision,* or *tylectomy*.

Lymph node dissection: Surgery that removes lymph nodes.

Magnetic resonance imaging (MRI): The use of magnetic signals to provide information on the internal makeup of breast tissue.

Mammogram: X-rays of the breast used to detect breast cancer and other breast diseases.

Margins: The amount of normal tissue that was removed with the tumor.

Mastectomy: Removal of the breast. A *simple mastectomy* removes the entire breast; a *radical mastectomy* removes the breast and the axillary lymph nodes, or the lymph nodes in the armpits.

Metabolic syndrome: A combination of risk factors such as high blood glucose, high blood pressure, and abdominal obesity, plus cholesterol problems like low HDL ("good"cholesterol), high LDL ("bad"cholesterol), and high triglycerides.

Metaplastic breast cancer: A rare type of invasive ductal cancer, with cells from other parts of the body such as the skin and bone found inside the tumor.

Metastatic breast cancer: Cancer that has spread to distant organs.

Microtubule inhibitors: Drugs that kill cancer by disrupting its cellular balance. This includes ixabepilone (Ixempra) and eribulin.

Mitogen-activated protein (MAP): A genetic pathway, or part of the body's communication system, that is in the majority of breast cancers; basal types have more of it

Neoadjuvant chemotherapy: Chemotherapy given before surgery.

Nottingham Histologic Score: A numeric rating of a tumor based on its "mitotic"count, or how rapidly it appears to be dividing and growing. A grade I tumor has between 1 and 5 points and is slow-growing. A grade II has between 6 and 7 points and is growing at a medium pace. A grade III is over 8 points and is rapidly growing. Triple-negative cancers tend to be grade III.

Oncotype DX: A genomic test that can predict the likelihood of recurrence in early stage invasive hormone-positive breast cancer. At present it cannot be used for hormone-negative cancers.

Overall survival: Survival after a specific amount of time. Deaths from all causes are accounted for, not just deaths from breast cancer.

p53: A tumor suppressor that can slow the growth of cancer by repairing the DNA.

Parabens: Chemicals in cosmetics and personal care products such lotions, makeup, and antiperspirants.

PARP1, or Poly (ADP-ribose) polymerase: A pathway the body uses to block the development of cancer cells.

PARP inhibitors: Drugs that block the Poly (ADP-ribose) polymerase pathway.

Partial response: Some disease remains in the body, but it has decreased by 30 percent or more in size or number of lesions after neoadjuvant therapy. While less positive than a complete response, partial response nevertheless shows that chemo has worked.

PET: Chemobiological therapy using an anthracycline, a taxane, and a platinum agent. Common regimens include Cisplatin, Epirubicin, and Paclitaxel.

Phthalates: Plastic compounds in baby powder, lotions, shampoo, and other personal care products.

Poorly differentiated: A tumor description that means it is high grade, or fast-growing.

Positive margins: Cancer that continues to the edge of the tissue taken during surgery.

Primary tumor: The original tumor at the site at which it first developed.

Progesterone: A hormone produced by the ovaries, the adrenal gland, and, during pregnancy, the placenta.

Progesterone-receptor-negative breast cancer: Cancer that lacks receptors for the hormone progesterone.

Radiation: Local treatment directly to the breast, using high-energy radiation to kill the cancer cells in the area that is irradiated.

Recurrence: The reappearance of cancer after remission.

Relapse-free survival: Survival after a specific time with no sign of disease; also called *disease-free survival.*

Relative risk: Risk based on your original diagnosis.

Salpingo-oophorectomy: Surgery to remove the ovaries and fallopian tubes.

Sentinel node dissection: A method of determining if cancer has spread to the lymph nodes.

Stable disease: The disease has remained unchanged in size and number of lesions. A decrease of less than 30 percent or a slight increase in size is generally considered stable disease.

Surgical biopsy, also called an excisional biopsy: Surgery that removes either the entire suspicious mass or a portion of it for study. Performed in an operating room under anesthesia. The tissue is then sent to pathology for testing.

Taxanes: Microtubule inhibitors and antimitotic agents that stop cancer cell division. These include paclitaxel (Taxol, Abraxane, and Apo-Paclitaxel), Docetaxel (Taxotere), and nab-paclitaxel (Abraxane).

Tamoxifen: An estrogen antagonist, or drug that blocks the effects of estrogen, and is given most often to premenopausal women with hormone-positive disease. Not recommended for hormone-negative or TNBC.

TAC: Chemotherapy using an anthracycline and an alkylating agent, plus a taxane administered concurrently. This is usually for aggressive breast cancers—large, locally advanced, or metastatic.

TC: Chemotherapy using a taxane plus an alkylating agent, usually Cytoxan.

Thermography: The use of infrared imaging to detect changes in breast cancer tissue.

Triple-negative breast cancer: Negative for estrogen and progesterone receptors and for Her2/neu. Also called *TNBC*.

Tumor size: A three-dimensional measurement of the invasive component.

Ultrasound: Test using sound waves that can analyze abnormalities found on a mammogram.

VEGF: Vascular endothelial growth factor, a protein that stimulates the development and growth of blood vessels.

VEGF inhibitor: A drug that starves the cancerous tumor by compromising its supply of blood, oxygen, and other nutrients. This includes bevacizumab (Avastin) and sorafenib (Nexavar).

Well differentiated: A tumor description that means it is low grade, or slow-growing; it looks more like normal cells.

Index